Healing Through Meeting

of related interest

Imagery and Symbolism in Counselling
William Stewart
ISBN 1 85302 350 7

Dictionary of Images and Symbols in Counselling
William Stewart
ISBN 1 85302 351 5

**Counselling Adult Survivors
of Child Sexual Abuse, Second edition**
Christiane Sanderson
ISBN 1 85302 252 7

The Listening Reader
Fiction and Poetry for Counsellors and Psychotherapists
Ben Knights
ISBN 1 85302 266 7

Not Too Late
Ageing and Psychotherapy
Ann Orbach
ISBN 1 85302 380 9

Healing Through Meeting

Martin Buber's Conversational
Approach to Psychotherapy

John C. Gunzburg

Foreword by Zena Burgess

Jessica Kingsley Publishers
London and Bristol, Pennsylvania

This book is dedicated to my mother, Eva Gunzburg, who loves to tell
stories, and to my father, Noah Gunzburg, who delights in listening to them.

The right of John C. Gunzburg to be identified as author of this work has been asserted
by him in accordance with the Copyright, Designs and Patents Act 1988.

First published in the United Kingdom in 1997 by
Jessica Kingsley Publishers Ltd
116 Pentonville Road
London N1 9JB, England
and
1900 Frost Road, Suite 101
Bristol, PA 19007, U S A

Copyright © 1997 John C. Gunzburg
Foreword copyright © 1997 Zena Burgess

Library of Congress Cataloging in Publication Data
A CIP catalogue record for this book is available from the Library of Congress

British Library Cataloguing in Publication Data
Gunzburg, John C.
Healing through meeting : Martin Buber's conversational
approach to psychotherapy
1. Psychotherapy 2. Psychotherapy – Practice 3. Conversation –
Psychological aspects
I. Title
616.8'914

ISBN 1-85302-375-2

Printed and Bound in Great Britain by
Cromwell Press, Melksham, Wiltshire

Contents

List of Figures and Tables

Acknowledgements

My appreciation goes to all clients whose stories have been shared in this text; to my academic soulmate, William Stewart, for introducing me to Jessica Kingsley; to my colleagues and the staff at the Hennessy Clinic – Charles, John A, John B, Zena, Harvey, Chris, Linda and Robyn – for their support and friendship; to Rabbi Yaacov Barber, with whom I continue to unravel the mysteries of Torah in a spirit of warm connection, and to my many friends at South Caulfield Hebrew Congregation, a vibrant, nourishing and frustrating network, and particularly to Claire and Julian Boymal for their love and care; to cousins Lottie and Heinz, parents-in-law Dennis and Edith, brother Ron, sister-in-law Paula, cousins Adrian, Linda, Jeremy and Benjy, brother-in-law Robert, his wife Ginette, niece Judith and nephew Asher, Aunts Esme and Nan, cousins Anna, Robert, Jeremy and Jessica, cousins Paul and Cindy, cousins Terry, Dina, Michal and Alon, for 'being there'; to McGraw-Hill for their permission to reprint material from Chapters 1, 15, 20, 21, 22, 23, 24, 25, 31, 32, 33, 35, 38, 43 of my previous book, *The Family Counselling Casebook* (McGraw-Hill, Sydney, 1991) and to Adis International for allowing me to print material from the (*Casebook, Keys to Effective Counselling*, and) *Therapeutic Encounters* series.

As always, my love goes to my wife Joy and daughters Rahel, Aviva and Penina for their patience and understanding during the composition of this book.

Foreword

I have known Dr John Gunzburg for nearly a decade and am delighted to provide you, the reader, with some introductory comments about this volume.

This book is as much about John Gunzburg's own journey as a therapist and a man in contemporary society, as about the stories and meanings co-created with his clients. Reflected in this volume is John's value that, for every client with whom he has worked, he considers it a deep privilege to have the opportunity to share their stories so personally and intimately.

Out of his clinical experience and research, John has written many papers and articles. This collection focuses on clients' search for meaning, often in the areas of relationships and recovery from abuse. Yet these topics are covered in a new and exciting manner.

John demonstrated his gift for story-telling in therapy in his first book, *The Family Counselling Casebook*. In this volume he uses the philosophy of Martin Buber, prose, metaphor, stories and poetry to illustrate the rich tapestry of his clients' lives and solutions to difficulties. Each of the stories told in this volume has relevance for everyday living and will resonate with your personal experience. Yet the book does not prescribe or offer advice.

This book will appeal to those people from many disciplines who have an interest in family therapy and counselling and to people interested in a variety of experience. The busy clinician can read part of this volume, or even a few pages, and gain ideas or strategies to deal with a similar situation. For those who learn from example, this is a helpful text.

It is my hope that by reading this work you will find the new ideas and learnings that occur will enrich your lives, as you will find courage and greater strength inspired by the stories told.

Zena Burgess,
Clinical Psychologist,
Swinburne University of Technology,
Melbourne, Australia.

Frontispiece

'Peekay,' he said, 'in this world are very few things made from logic alone. It is illogical for a man to be too logical. Some things we must just let stand. The mystery is more important than any possible explanation'. He paused for a moment and tapped his fingers on the edge of the keyboard. 'The searcher after truth must search with humanity. Ruthless logic is the sign of a limited mind. The truth can only add to the sum of what you know, while a harmless mystery left unexplored often adds to the meaning of life. When a truth is not so important, it is better left as a mystery.'

Bryce Courtenay, *The Power of One*, p.325.

Preface

When a person sings and cannot lift their voice, and another comes and sings with them, another who can lift their voice, then the first will be able to lift their voice too. That is the secret of the bond between spirit and spirit. (Rabbi Pinhas of Koretz in Buber 1947, p.126)

The eyes of the Yehudi flamed. 'What is it that you have learned in Lublin,' he cried, 'if you have not learned this, that each has his own way of serving. Did not Rabbi David tell me how once upon a time disciples of a famous Zaddik came, after the Zaddik's death, to the Rabbi of Lublin. They arrived in the evening and found him standing on the road where he was pronouncing the *sanctification of the moon,* which was just emerging from the clouds. They observed at once that his custom in regard to the ceremony differed somewhat from that of their late teacher. They nudged each other. When, later, they entered the house of the Rabbi, he greeted them and said: 'What kind of a God would He be, who has but a single way of serving Him!'

Another student had sprung to his feet and now lifted his hand. 'What have you in mind, Yissachar Baer?', he was asked. Slowly and solemnly he answered: 'It is true; it is true indeed. I myself besought the Rabbi to show me the way of service. The answer he gave was: 'There is none such. It will not do to tell one's comrade what way he is to pursue. There is a way of serving God by study, another of serving Him by prayer; one by deeds of loving-kindness toward one's fellows; there is a way to be pursued by fasting and there is one to be pursued by eating. And all these are right ways to the service of God. But each man is to observe well toward which one of these ways his heart inclines him. Thereupon, he is to be active upon that way with all his might.' (Buber 1981, pp.33–4)

In his Preface to *Tales of the Hasidim*, Martin Buber writes:

One of the most vital aspects of the Hasidic movement is that the Hasidim tell one another stories about their leaders, their 'Zaddikim'. Great things had happened, the Hasidim had been present, they had seen them, and so they felt called upon to relate and bear witness to them. The words used to describe these experiences were more than mere words; they transmitted what had happened to coming generations, and with such actuality that the words in themselves became events. And since they serve to perpetuate holy events, they bear the consecration of holy deeds. It is told that the 'Seer' of Lublin once saw a pillar of light rise out of a klaus; when he entered he saw Hasidim telling one another about their Zaddikim. According to Hasidic belief, the primeval light of God poured into the Zaddikim; from them it poured into their works, and from these into the words of the Hasidim who relate them. The Baal Shem, the founder of Hasidism, is supposed to have said that when a Hasid spoke in praise of the Zaddikim, this was equivalent to dwelling on the mystery of the divine Chariot which Ezekiel once saw. And a Zaddik of the fourth generation, Rabbi Mendel of Rymanov, a friend of the 'Seer', added an explanation: 'For the Zaddikim *are* the chariot of God'.[1]

But story is more than a mere reflection. The holy essence it testifies to lives on in it. The miracle that is told, acquired new force; power that was once active, is propagated in the living word and continues to be active – even after generations.

A rabbi, whose grandfather had been a disciple of the Baal Shem, was asked to tell a story. 'A story', he said, 'must be told in such a way that it constitutes help in itself'. And he told: 'My grandfather was lame. Once they asked him to tell a story about his teacher. And he related how the holy Baal Shem used to hop and dance while he prayed. My grandfather rose as he spoke, and he was so swept away by his story that he himself began to hop and dance to show how the master had done. From that hour on he was cured of his lameness. That's the way to tell a story!'

My great-grandfather was Rav Schneur Zalman Gunzburg of Minsk. Of his published writings, only a few Hebrew poems remain – so mystical in their content that they are difficult to comprehend – but his descendants tell stories in a variety of contexts. My first cousin, Adrian Gunzburg, is an internation-ally-renowned writer on steam locomotives. His sister, Darrelyn, is an

1   Quoted from Midrash Genesis Rabba LXXXII 7 cf. Rashi on Genesis 17:22.

award-winning playwright. Another first cousin, Eddie Gunzburg, is a journalist and his son, Danny, is a poet. Our mutual cousin, Medad Schiff, is a retired newspaper editor and his son, Agur, has recently published his first book of short stories, written in Hebrew. I write my therapeutic tales. Each of us, in our own way, tells the stories of his or her experiences, and the experiences of those whom we encounter, within our fields of interaction.

It is my privilege to compose this book in honour of our common ancestor, Rav Schneur Zalman Gunzburg of Minsk. In Section One, an introduction to the life and ideas of Martin Buber creates a philosophical framework within which to have a therapeutic conversation. Section Two further examines the power of story. It touches briefly on a number of concepts from differing therapeutic frameworks and illustrates how those ideas can be conveyed to clients through the telling of story, and when to tell them. The third section examines how Buber's philosophical themes are contained, under other names, within the frameworks of a number of other explorers of mind and illustrates how to construct tales of empowerment. It includes a selection of stories, each demonstrating how Buber's ideas weave throughout the therapeutic conversation in a diversity of situations. This whole book is presented in the Hasidic tradition, except that the tales I have written in it are not composed about my 'leaders' but, rather, about my clients – they who have told me their stories, shared their struggles and taught me their wisdom. I have tried to relate their accounts in such a way that their stories 'constitute help' in themselves. My hope is that readers will be 'swept away' by the stories; that they will start to resonate to the rhythms within the telling and flow through the discordant passages towards the more harmonious resolutions that evolve. In so doing, I hope that readers will understand more about the process of therapeutic dialogue that can lead to healing, integration and empowerment for both client and therapist.

Section One

'Orthodox, Western psychology has dealt very poorly with the spiritual side of our nature, choosing either to ignore its existence or to label it pathological. Yet much of the agony of our time stems from a spiritual vacuum. Our culture, our psychology, has ruled out our spiritual nature, but the cost of this attempted suppression is enormous. If we want to find ourselves, our spiritual side, it's imperative for us to look at the psychologies that deal with it. (Tart 1976, p.5)[1]

Introduction

Before examining Martin Buber's ideas in detail, it is necessary to consider the existential, phenomenological and humanistic philosophies within which his concepts are grounded.

Existentialism

This philosophy focuses on the uniqueness and isolation of individual experience in a seemingly indifferent and even hostile universe. It asserts that human existence is unexplainable and that humans are responsible for the consequences of their own acts towards themselves and towards others. We are real only to ourselves and we are our own judgments. Ultimate reality is rejected and objectivity is considered an illusion. Truth is regarded as a personal realization, unique to each person, and it cannot be hardened into dogma. To be able to grasp what is not the case, as well as what is, is considered the basis of possibility. To claim that one is bound to do something, or could not help it, is considered self-deception. We all choose our own morality and some existentialists believe that personal relations can never be other than a struggle for power. (Stewart 1992, p.80)

Buber considers that we are free to be reconciled to God.

---

1   This section was presented in abbreviated form in *Psychotherapy in Australia 1*, 3, November 1996, 33–8.

Phenomenology

Phenomenology is a school of philosophy that arose in the early years of the present century. It is the study of all human experience as free as possible from presupposition or bias. Phenomenology is the basic method of existentialism. Phenomenologists limit their study to conscious experiences without trying to elicit underlying hypothetical causes. The data they produce are formulated from the other person's point of view.

Phenomenologists as a rule reject the idea of the unconscious. They believe we can learn more about human nature by studying how people view themselves and their world than we can by observing their actions. In that phenomenologists are more concerned with internal mental processes and the inner life and experience of individuals – self-concept, feelings of self-esteem and self-awareness – than with behaviour, they have certain similarity to cognitivists.

Phenomenologists believe that we are free agents, that we are not acted upon by forces beyond our control, but that we have a great degree of control over our destiny i.e. the issue of free will versus determinism.

Most humanistic approaches, with their emphasis on self-actualization, are grounded in phenomenology. A phenomenological approach concentrates on what is happening now. Most personality theories look at a person from the outside; phenomenology attempts to enter a person's own psychological experience, to try to understand what something means to that person. (Stewart 1992, p.202)

Humanism

Humanism is a philosophy which attaches importance to humankind and human values. Although fundamentally eclectic, there are common themes within humanism. Central are the ideas of personal growth, human potential, responsibility, and self direction. Human experience is considered to be a lifelong education which can lead to full emotional functioning. There is recognition of the need to learn, or to relearn, what play and joy are about. There is appreciation of a person's spirituality, with an acknowledgment of human capacity for altered states of consciousness. Intense personal experiences are considered to alter radically a person's attitudes to self and others, and through such experiences, a unity of the human and natural can be achieved. Such experiences can lead to a person becoming completely independent and totally responsible for their thoughts and actions. (Stewart 1992, p.113)

Martin Buber was a Hasidic existentialist philosopher who believed in the connection of all living things. He had a passionate interest in the relationships between people, how they experienced their world and how they made meaning out of what they were experiencing. For Buber, experiences – love, fear, hatred, trust, friendliness, despair – were not simply words and abstract notions but expressions of what people were experiencing about their world and about themselves. It was Buber's contention that the human purpose of life was to experience the world. Humans were not dwellers in abstract concepts and theoretical realms. Rather, they were to plunge deep into the experience. To experience a facet of the world was like trying on a piece of clothing, checking its fit, examining it, talking about it and sharing it with others. During this process of sharing with others, experiences could be explored, defined and re-defined until they were clarified and better understood.

Although trained as an anthropologist and philosopher, Buber's ideas always contained a spiritual aspect. Buber believed in the principles of Hasidism: that the world is a whole, that all its parts are connected and interacting and that harmony and integration within the world is achievable. For Buber, the process of attaining balance and integration was through conversation. Buber's basic idea was that, in conversation between two people, there is no self and other, no us and them, no subject and object; there are two people in conversation who share a connected human experience which they are both struggling to comprehend.

> We do exist, Yeshaya; that is not a delusion. True it is that we are mere creatures, frailer than any other creatures. Not for nothing were we formed of clay. Yet is that not a mighty matter when we think of the Hand of the Potter which kneaded our clay? The imprint of its fingers are visible upon its handiwork. Nor is this all. There is more. He breathed His breath into us, and if we are able to live from within outward as no other created thing may do, it is because His breath enables us to do so. How fair and marvellous it is, Yeshaya, to know at the same time that all images are naught before Him, yet to be able to speak of Him in images drawn from the image of us, of our mortal being – to be able to do so, to be forced to do so, but also to be permitted to do so, because in His image did He create us! His breath! His countenance! His glance!

> Yeshaya let an interval lapse before he spoke again.

'I love your enthusiasm,' he said, 'and yet I dread it too. I cannot but remember how in your boyhood you were often so exhausted by prayer you seemed to swoon. Yet out of ecstasy all one can draw is a recurrent dying again – never a true life. And therefore I want to tell you another thing before I say farewell. Often now, as in your boyhood, you wait to pray until enthusiasm overcomes you. That is not the right way. We do not pray according to the inspiration of the individual heart. We join an ordering of the word of prayer which generations of our fathers organically built. We subordinate ourselves to and within this ordering not as this *I* or this *you*, but as part of that congregation in the act of prayer with which you and I are integrated. What your single heart bids you tell your Creator you can utter in the solitariness of your waking at dawn or in your lonely walks. But the order of prayer has its place and its appointed times, which you should respect.' (Buber 1981, pp.101–2)

As is often the case, Buber's early experiences were formative on his thinking in adult life. Born into a Jewish Viennese family in 1878, his parents divorced three years later. The youthful Buber had no connection with his mother and this separation seems to have had considerable impact on him. Whilst still a toddler, a young girl much older than Buber had declared that 'she [his mother] will never come back' (Buber 1973, p.18). Buber developed an idea out of this remembered episode which he called *mismeeting* – an event which occurs when one person is not fully available towards another – reflecting Buber's experience of his mother's absence.

The presence of Buber's paternal grandparents, with whom he stayed until he was fourteen, also had a marked influence on him. The grandfather was well versed in Talmudic knowledge whereas the grandmother's interest lay in secular literature. The grandfather offered Buber the information that he was obliged to know as a Jew whereas the grandmother risked sharing with Buber 'other' texts that Jews were not permitted to read. So, although both encouraged Buber's intellectual growth, it was the grandmother who taught him to value the difference between, and the diversity within, the sacred and the secular; that both encompassed descriptions about the world that were genuine. One could read books both holy and mundane, reflect on the material, transcend the content of their text and inspirit oneself. It was this process of reflection that enabled one to rise above the content, that created a wholeness and unification of experience, a continuum of reading, reflecting, reading, reflecting…

Buber's father, with whom he stayed after the age of fourteen, left a different mark on him. As Buber describes it, his father's teaching 'did not derive at all from mind' (Buber 1973, p.22). Instead, he delighted in a communion with nature, a sense of ecology that embraced human society as well as all things natural.

During his teenage years, Buber studied Hasidism, rationalism, and existentialism, continuing to read and reflect. However, the process for Buber gradually changed. Rather than concentrating on reading, he started to throw himself into a series of experiences, taking time out to withdraw himself from each one to reflect on its consequences. He decided that the sole purpose of human exploration was the examination of self-existence – its wonders, dilemmas, life and death – and finding of hope in the midst of despair:

'I am about to die,' said the man in the bed.

In this instant, with a glance of the almost unknown man upon him, the Yehudi became aware of the fact that suddenly the fruit of his sufferings had ripened. .

'Assuredly you will die,' said he, and laughed into the other's eyes, 'but not necessarily right away.'

'I shall die soon,' said the man.

'No mortal can know the time of his death with such exactness', answered the Yehudi. 'I know what you mean,' he continued, 'your limbs and your very entrails feel sore; you are tired to death and you think that any little extra blow, a tug at your shoulder, a cold breath on the back of your neck, is bound to finish you. But all this has only the character of a question addressed to the sufferer, whether he is willing that his end come to him. If he summons his last strength to utter a "No", or, rather, if he rouses himself to a beseeching of the Eternal over the head of the Angel who asks the question – then it may well be that the hand which is stretched out toward him falls again.'

'Not so,' said the man in a beseeching voice, 'I know that my hour approaches.'

'Whence do you know that?'

'I know it.'

'Forget what you think you know,' the Yehudi demanded with repressed power, 'and turn your face to the Lord of Life.' The sick man was silent. But he who had undertaken to draw him back to life observed that something had come to pass. Those eyes left his own and closed; the lips met tranquilly; the emaciated body seemed for the first time in many days to relax. Minutes passed. The drops of a gentle rain of June pattered against the window panes. The clock on the wall struck the hour. The Yehudi stood still and remained with a gesture of helpfulness where he had been standing. Again the hour struck. The sick man opened his eyes and lips. His glance was lost in the distance. 'Blessed art Thou, King of the Universe,' he whispered. The remainder of the blessing was not audible.

'Go down to the tap room,' said the Yehudi to the man's son, 'and ask them to give you a jug of mead.' The youth looked at him in dismay and went. 'Now we will drink *l'hayyim* – to a good life – to each other,' said the Yehudi and put the jug to his lips. The sick man drank a deep draught. Then he drank another and fell asleep at once. A mild perspiration gathered on his forehead. The clock struck two. The Yehudi sat down by the side of the bed and kept his vigil until dawn. By that time it was clear to him that life had gained a victory. (Buber 1981, pp.132–3)

These themes which Buber has given us: that people share a connected human experience which they are struggling to comprehend; that conversation occurs between two persons who experience themselves, each other and their world as subjects, not objects; that there is a diversity in life to be celebrated and a difference to be respected; and that the process of life consists of plunging into an experience and then reflecting on that experience, can be regarded as the framework in which the therapeutic conversation occurs. For Buber, when therapist[2] and client *meet*, that encounter is not as therapist/subject and client/object, but as existential equals meeting within the conversational space between them. It was this concept of *the between* that was crucial to Buber's philosophy. The genuineness of the therapeutic conversation is not the responsibility of the therapist or client, it is in the nature of the connectedness that lies between both, within the *meeting* of both. It is not the therapist's concern to 'be genuine' or 'sincere' or 'empathetic' in some contrived fashion. Instead, the client forwards a problem and it is the therapist's responsibility to ensure that an environment occurs in which *meeting* can take place and a new facet of the problem can be explored. Often the client cannot describe his or her dilemma and the

---

2   Throughout this book I have used the term *therapy* as the shortened form of *psychotherapy* to acknowledge psyche as *soul*, and therapy as *taking care of*. Therapist and client have by now become communally recognized terms, though arguably so, for one who offers and one who seeks therapy, respectively.

therapist can offer a conversational space in which the problem can be named, experienced, defined and re-defined. This process is illustrated in the following case.[3]

Case 1A: Lunch[4]

Cal, 35 years, and Sylvie, 31 years, had hit a lull in their marriage. Both fully occupied in their careers and effective in their role as parents to their two pre-adolescent children, they reported little shared enjoyment between themselves during the previous year or so. They rarely went out together without their children and both felt as if they had stopped caring for each other. 'What would have to happen', I asked, 'to let each other know that you cared?' Cal replied that he would like Sylvie to make his lunch each morning for him, before he left for work. Sylvie said that she would like more time alone with Cal, spent in conversation. By the next session, two weeks later, Sylvie had invited, and taken, Cal out to a restaurant lunch!

Discussion

By encouraging this couple to define exactly what the word 'care' meant to each of them, they came up with a solution which tended to both their needs and instigated a small change in their mode of relating. A basic event that the therapeutic conversation aims to achieve is illustrated here. Cal wanted 'A' (Sylvie to tend to his needs more and make him lunch). Sylvie wanted 'B' (Cal to tend to her needs more and to talk to her). Their solution achieved a synthesis. It provided both 'A' and 'B' in a manner in which they could give to each other without the feeling of 'giving in' to one another. Importantly, it was Cal and Sylvie's solution that was effective. The therapist's task can be regarded as not to provide answers but to facilitate a process whereby participants can clarify what they are saying to each other and come up with their own resolution. Such a clarification takes place during an encounter which Buber would call *meeting*.

For Buber, 'All real living is meeting', (1958, p.11). For therapist and client, conversation can be considered as reflecting the world of 'real living' outside the therapy room. So, the effective therapeutic conversation can be regarded as containing elements of 'real living' that occurs in other arenas.

---

3 All the case studies presented in this book have the permission of the clients involved. In all cases, names and other identifying details have been changed to preserve confidentiality. If, perchance, readers recognize any identity, the author requests that readers take care to be silent and protect confidentiality to esteem the courage of those clients who have shared their wisdom with us.

4 This case was originally presented in *Patient Management 14*, 8, August 1990, 101–8.

Two of these elements that are essential to Buber's philosophy are the concepts of I–It and I–Thou:

> To Man the world is twofold, in accordance with his twofold attitude.
>
> The attitude of Man is twofold, in accordance with the twofold nature of the primary words that he speaks. The primary words are not isolated words, but combined words.
>
> The one primary word is the combination of 'I–Thou'.
>
> The other primary word is the combination 'I–It'.
>
> Primary words do not signify things but they intimate relations.
>
> Primary words do not describe something that might exist independently of them but, being spoken, they bring about existence. Primary words are spoken from the being. (Buber 1958, pp.3–4)

Case 1B: The boss[5]

Howard, 49 years, expressed feelings of guilt and fear of criticism from his boss. He found himself incapable of forwarding reasonable complaints about problems with his workmates or of being able to approach his boss and request a long-overdue pay rise. 'I am not good enough and the boss will sack me', said Howard, even though, as departmental manager, he had increased company productivity within his section by 30 per cent during the previous year. Howard had displayed episodes of violent temper in the past and said that, as a youth, he had almost strangled a school-fellow. 'The headmaster had to drag me off him', he said. Our therapeutic conversation took up this theme of Howard's previous violation of his school-fellow. Howard's guilt was re-framed as 'responsible concern'. It was a part of Howard that could be regarded as protecting him, avoiding undue conflict and possible violent behaviour towards his boss and enabling Howard to maintain his employment. Howard was then encouraged, via role play (Howard playing the boss and the therapist playing Howard), to explore appropriate ways of encountering his boss. He learnt new behaviours and commenced asserting himself successfully, both with the therapist and at work.

Discussion

Howard can be regarded as viewing his relationship with his boss within Buber's I–It position. Howard appeared to see himself as the 'helpless

---

5   This case was originally presented in *Patient Management 13*, 7, July 1989, 103–11.

employee' unable to forward his needs to a 'cruel and insensitive' boss. He did not acknowledge his own competence or the boss's ability to recognize Howard's worth to the company. In this position, Howard was constantly fearful of the boss's reprimands and he experienced guilt for his perceived failings. The therapeutic conversation emphasized Howard's genuine concern for others through his restraint on his temper and new assertive skills were explored through the use of psychodrama. Howard tried these out successfully in his workplace. Eventually, Howard may come to realize that, in this different relationship with his boss, both are subject to the vicissitudes of life and develop an understanding towards him – an example of Buber's I–Thou position.

Buber considered that there were two existential positions within conversation: the I–It position – in which people considered one another as an It, an object, without particular regard for the complexities of their personhood – and the I–Thou position – in which people regarded each other as subjects and struggled to understand the complexities of their personhood. It is not inherently 'bad' to enter an I–It position; we often do it when we buy a dozen eggs from the grocer or when we accept the communally nominated roles of 'therapist' and 'client'. Such nominations enable us to understand easily our relationship with others and our initial purpose in meeting them. The position only becomes problematical when one person constantly views the other as an object in his or her field of experience, to be used or exploited without regard for that other's personhood. Buber considered that most of our existence was lived within the I–It position and that the I–Thou position only occurred infrequently during moments of intimacy and connection. 'The Thou meets one through Grace – it is not found by seeking.' (Buber 1958, p.11) And therein lies the therapeutic dilemma: the client usually commences therapy with the therapist in the I–It position, with both having some understanding of what they expect from each other, but *meeting* will only occur within the I–Thou position, which often occurs spontaneously and cannot be willed. Therapist and client can only hope to *meet*, never demand or will it of each other.

Case 1C: Creative relating[6]

Bess, 27 years, complained of constant depression and loss of confidence. A part-time journalist, she had been unable to work for many months and bemoaned her lack of creative drive. Bess had been involved in an affair with Dan, a sculptor, for the previous six years. Dan, who had been living with

---

6   This case was originally presented in *Patient Management 13*, 7, July 1989, 103–11.

Meg during this time, had promised to leave her for Bess when their affair had commenced but this had not eventuated. Bess' description of her mother had been that of 'an efficient, dominating, discounting woman', and of her father, 'a depressed, isolated man always suffering migraines'. She suspected that their marriage of 29 years had been largely unrewarding. During the first months of therapy, with Bess attending twice weekly, I endeavoured to model a different male–female connection with Bess from that which she had experienced with her father and Dan. Rather than the 'clinging, support me, don't leave me' attitude of those men who were having problems within their own marriages, I believe I established clear boundaries, a sense of equity, sharing of adult life experiences, respect and the right to privacy. We discussed the painful nature of triangular relationships, the development of self, handling of primitive drives, the blessing and curse of creativity – with its compulsive urge to synthesize and reorganize experiences – and peer interactions. The sessions themselves developed very much into an existential dialogue between equals. I drew Bess an illustration of what I understood the process within this therapy to be (see Figure 1.1).

Bess is now in the process of leaving Dan and engaging with others within a wider social network. She has commenced teaching her craft at night-school and has recommenced freelancing. Therapy lasted a little over a year in duration.

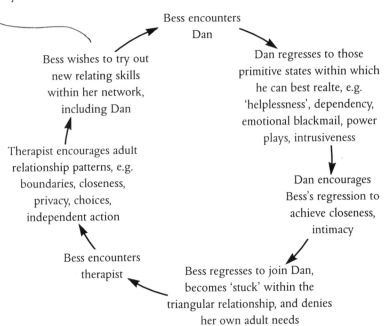

Bess encounters
Dan

Bess wishes to try out
new relating skills
within her network,
including Dan

Dan regresses to those
primitive states within which
he can best realte, e.g.
'helplessness', dependency,
emotional blackmail, power
plays, intrusiveness

Therapist encourages adult
relationship patterns, e.g.
boundaries, closeness,
privacy, choices,
independent action

Dan encourages
Bess's regression to
achieve closeness,
intimacy

Bess encounters
therapist

Bess regresses to join Dan,
becomes 'stuck' within the
triangular relationship, and denies
her own adult needs

Figure 1.1 John's drawing for Bess

Discussion

Bess came to therapy with depression, loss of confidence and lack of creative drive. Early exploration enabled her to recognize her symptoms and take practical measures to care for herself on 'off' days. As therapy progressed, Bess discovered the context in which her depression was occurring: the triangular relationship with Dan and Meg. We considered the roles that Bess valued as important to her: living up to her mother's expectations and her desire to support Dan in his career as 'young, struggling artist'. The mother and Dan could both be regarded as relating to Bess within an I–It position: demanding that Bess tend to their requirements at the expense of her own. Bess's need for intimate contact with another creative companion could be considered as an example of an I–Thou stance: she desired that she and her partner meet within the creative realm to grow and develop together. The therapist took up this theme and also wished to meet Bess within the creative arena. He offered her the diagram in an attempt to integrate intrapsychic and interactional processes in Bess' life. The therapist and Bess can be regarded as conversing within an I–Thou position: using the drawing, the therapist shared his skills with Bess – his ability to synthesize a solution from a number of perspectives and his capacity to stand outside the problem to see a specific part within the whole pattern. The therapist encouraged Bess to use these skills herself, re-examine her position and interrupt the cyclic pattern of interactions involving herself and Dan (I–It) and herself and the therapist (I–Thou). Subsequently, Bess chose a number of contexts within which she could achieve relationships within an I–Thou position: successfully completing therapy, increasing contact with peers who nourished and stimulated her healthy growth, teaching her craft to the next generation and pursuing her writing. Hopefully, Bess' own sense of wholeness will continue to be enhanced as she seeks progressive I–Thou relationships, rather than regressive I–It contacts, to become an effective participant within the wider community.

Another area which Buber explored is the capacity of people to reconcile contrary positions within their experiences. Much of Western thinking is involved in an either/or attitude; that no two objects can occupy the same space. In relationships, this is often translated into the view that no two beliefs can occupy the same conversational space – frequently leading to opposing stances: 'either my belief or your belief' and, even more frequently when there is conflict, 'only my belief, never your belief'. Buber was concerned with achieving a both/and attitude during conversation, in creating a space in which both therapist's and client's beliefs were to be spoken and heard. Buber alleges that: 'According to the logical conception of truth, only one of two contraries can be true but, in reality of life as one lives it, they are inseparable' (Buber 1948, p.17; Friedman 1960, p.3). 'The unity of the contraries is the mystery at the innermost core of dialogue' (Buber 1948, p.17). Therapy offers an opportunity where the therapist's and client's beliefs can be aired and a connection between them discovered, as is illustrated in Cases 1D and 1E.

Case 1D: Intriguing the analytic side[7]

Bernadette, 36 years, felt that her life was over. A secondary school mathematics teacher for twelve years, she had been married recently, for the first time, to Daniel, 37 years, an accountant. Seven months previously she had been a joyful bride, yet now her world was in pieces.

The crisis had commenced when Danny, a senior student, had been openly rude and disruptive in class. Bernadette had expelled Danny from the classroom, only to find him poking his head through the windows and provoking other class members into disarray. She had lost control. Now, ten weeks later, Bernadette was 'off on Workcare' and did not know which way her direction led.

On further enquiry, I found that Bernadette (originally a native of middle Europe) appeared to be well qualified, having gained a masters degree with a major in psychology. She had developed several training programmes for ethnic students (these had been cut due to lack of funding) and had written numerous articles on education. Bernadette said that she was enjoying her marriage with Daniel, whom she described as laid-back and fun-loving. She termed herself as intense and sensitive, a real analytical thinker.

I commented on Bernadette's dedication to her vocation and the enormous effort and energy that she had put into her career. I suggested that perhaps it was now time for a change and asked if she wanted to work at a different level. Rather than disseminating information to students, she might wish, at this stage of her life, to help organize, via research and/or administration, the structures in which teaching occurred. We discussed the different ways of gaining knowledge about our world. Sometimes we learnt in an analytic, rational fashion whereas at other times we used a holistic, synthetic process. I remarked how I, as a trained violinist, and Bernadette, as a skilled mathematician, both needed discipline to be effective in these talents, using both intellectual and holistic means of learning. Bernadette's articles had been a beautifully collated series of events, dates and places,

---

7   This case was originally presented in the *Newsletter of the Victorian Association of Family Therapists,* November 1989, 10–12.

constructed with precision. I offered her a paper on family therapy (Gunzburg 1991) that illustrated the holistic nature of human interaction and asked her to write a commentary on it, part of which is reproduced below:

> This paper reminded me of what life in general is all about; namely, a 'puzzle'. That is, each individual is trying to find the 'missing bits'. In so doing, one can subsequently piece them together. Consequently, one is able to establish a much more rewarding, fulfilling and richer personal existence.
>
> The ability to do this piecing together and find the missing bits is very much dependent on a person's abilities/goals/ambitions; past experiences and feelings; and capacities to resolve problems/conflicts. Furthermore, it reflects the person's level of motivation and desire to make this work and their ability to analyze problems and logically, step by step, seek plausible solutions. One needs to 'stand back' and take stock of the situation, to become personally detached and objective. This applies very much to real life. If one is involved in a problem situation, one needs to stand back and unemotionally and logically sort things out.

Discussion

Bernadette came to therapy biased towards using the analytical side of her personality. She had indicated that she wanted to marry Daniel, an easy-going, good-humoured partner. Danny, the practical-joking student, had disrupted her sense of control and induced crises in both classroom and psyche. Therapy proceeded (twice weekly over two months) by:

1. Affirming Bernadette's dedication to her work.

2. Discussing how *both* analytic *and* holistic ways of learning are essential to achieve discipline in varying fields (e.g. music, mathematics). Bernadette's discipline had been challenged by Danny and was now in tatters. The discipline underlying Bernadette's mathematical and writing capabilities was highlighted as a resource.

3. Commenting on the complementarity between Bernadette (academic, serious) and Daniel (leisurely, fun-loving).

4. Encouraging Bernadette's creativity; intriguing her analytic side in writing a commentary on the holistic nature of therapy and human interaction. This she did, extending the information gleaned to her own life experiences and finding some of her own resources – the ability to stand back and view the whole, rather than the specific.

Bernadette actively sought different employment in a research administration field; and, she became pregnant and was delighted about this! Three years later, Bernadette chose to be the full-time mother of two daughters.

Case 1E: Structuring the holistic side[8]

Jason, 61 years, was a lively, energetic man who bubbled about and irritated his wife and two adult children immensely with his interjections and disorganized behaviour. Jason hoarded magazines and his study and bedroom were absolute shambles. His wife slept in a separate bedroom.

Thinking to introduce a technique that might calm him down, I suggested: 'Would you take some time to stop your buzziness and practice an hour's relaxation each evening? I have an exercise that I could teach you'. Jason ceased his chatter, thought for a moment, then responded: 'I will reflect on it'. A pause ensued, then much laughter issued from us both; in reflecting, Jason had stared to quieten down.

Jason continued to relax and tell his story. He had collected several thousand articles, magazines and papers in his home over the decades. I enquired as to the date of the first item collected and Jason said that he could not remember this detail. He was employed as a librarian and offered a statement that he was researching material for a proposed book. Jason had brought me a poem that he had published several years earlier. I commented that perhaps Jason was a creative personality who had become stuck within his own process and drew for him a diagram (see Figure 1.2). I regard a creative personality as gathering data from the environment (using his/her analytic skills) then entering a period of disorganization where information is taken apart internally and examined (using both analytic and synthetic skills interchangeably, a state which often resembles confusion to outsiders). Finally, there is a creative expression of the reorganized information (using largely synthetic skills) within the individual's chosen medium: art, poetry, prose, music, sculpture, photography, dance, etc. It seemed a pity that Jason appeared to be expending so much energy within the gathering/disorganization phases of the cycle that there was none left to express himself and communicate his experiences to others. We agreed that he was overloaded with information and Jason contracted to clear out all articles more than two years old. He made a commitment to achieve this at the rate of ten papers daily.

---

8   This case was originally presented in the *Newsletter of the Victorian Association of Family Therapists,* November 1989, 10–12.

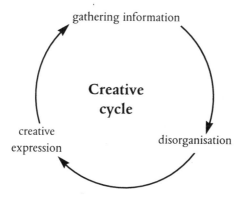

gathering information

Creative cycle

creative
expression

disorganisation

Figure 1.2 John's drawing for Jason

I shared with Jason that I was writing this story and requested his permission to use it in an educational paper. I wondered why I had chosen to call him Jason in the story. We talked about the mythical hero searching for the golden fleece and I said that I, too, was searching for a finish to this account of his case. Perhaps he would come up with the conclusion to his quest. Below is his response:

End of the quest

In his mind's eye, childhood shimmered sweetly;
There he sits...the sad old frustrated man.
He hunted for the golden fleece, they say,
Went with Jason to that fabled isle;
But his case is different,
No glory of discovery for him,
For his family suffered through his absence from home,
And so completely experienced the lack before his return
That wife was overcome with resentment of soul,
And children were gone...spirits flown away to lands unknown...
Now he sits there, his quest unfulfilled; an isolate alone...

After this, Jason and I were able to spend several sessions sharing his grief over past losses: his infertility (the children having been adopted), missed employment opportunities, his current sexual impotence and marriage dissolution. Seven months' after commencement of weekly therapy, Jason and his wife negotiated and completed their divorce, the study was half cleared of journals and Jason was contemplating his future as a single man. Three years later, Jason has retired, he has cordial relations with his children and contributes articles regularly to a local journal.

Discussion

Jason presented as a person with no emotional discipline and few organizational skills. Therapy aimed to:

1. Engage Jason and offer some relaxation tools to enable him to calm himself down.

2. Discover whether his hoarding had been triggered by some past traumatic event.

3. Reframe his confusion and disorganization within the 'creative process', thus giving Jason a conceptual structure.

4. Give Jason a practical framework within which he could clear the unfinished business of his life (i.e. a routine to tidy his study).

5. Encourage him to develop skills to contemplate the emotional leftovers from the past and his life ahead; in his poem, Jason expresses the enormous sense of loss underlying his 'manic' activity. He is able to grieve and then hope towards an easier future.

The human interactional world can be considered as containing contrary factors – analytic/synthetic; rational/intuitive; reductive-into-parts/holistic – and an imbalance between such factors can be regarded as disturbing to our emotional well-being and our communal life. The analytic/synthetic dichotomy is only one way of regarding such contraries. Chinese traditional practitioners talk of Yin and Yang (Wilhelm 1967) whereas Western religions mention the spiritual and the mundane (Frankl 1970). Freudians pay obeisance to the unconscious/conscious (Freud 1960) whereas Jungians heed the anima/animus (Jacobi 1973). Family therapists deal with enmeshed/disengaged families (Minuchin 1974) and regard communication patterns as digital or metaphoric (Gunzburg 1994). Erik Erikson (1968) defined various stages of psychological development in the individual at which certain contraries needed to be reconciled before progression to a subsequent psychological stage was possible: that is, within the first few years of life – basic trust/mistrust, autonomy/shame and initiative/guilt; within adolescence – industry/inferiority and identity/identity diffusion; within young adulthood – intimacy/isolation; within maturity – generativity/stagnation and ego-integrity/despair. Thus, non-attainment of basic trust in the initial stage of life could be regarded as leading to an adult troubled by mistrust of the wider world in later life. Those who had not been encouraged to take initiative in their kindergarten years could be considered to be frustrated by guilt from reaching later goals. Therapists invite their clients to reconcile these polarities in a number of ways (see Table 1.1).

Table 1.1: Ways in which therapists can invite
their clients to reconcile polarities

Polarities to be reconciled	Invitations to clients to reconcile their polarities
Basic trust/mistrust	Therapists can provide a confidential, reliable and regular service that is not financially onerous. Therapists can imagine the real of their clients' world: what has fostered their lack of safety? Therapists can offer clients acceptance, empathy, warmth, encouragement and affirmation. Therapists can invite clients to meet and enter into a genuine dialogue with them.
Autonomy/shame	Therapists can imagine the real of their clients' world: what is the basis of their sense of shame? Therapists can create a space for clients to tell their story freely, without qualification.
Initiative/guilt	Therapists can imagine the real of their clients' world: what is engendering their sense of guilt? Therapists can invite clients to explore the attitudes of people within their family of origin, and social contexts, who contributed to the development of the guilt. This may involve naming any abusers of the clients.
Industry/inferiority	Therapists can imagine the real of their clients' world: what is leading to their feelings of inferiority? Therapists can invite clients to participate in skills-training activities, assertiveness, emotional expression, rational thinking and usage of creative outlets, such as composing letters which contest any abuse.
Identity/identity diffusion	Therapists can imagine the real diffusion of their clients' world: what is influencing their experience of identity diffusion? Therapists can invite clients to break free from parental control, to regulate sexual and aggressive drives and to create meaning out of their lives. Such invitations can confirm clients in developing a stable sense of self that remains the same no matter how their lives progress.

Table 1.1: Ways in which therapists can invite their clients to reconcile polarities (continued)

Polarities to be reconciled	Invitations to clients to reconcile their polarities
Intimacy/isolation	Therapists can imagine the real of their clients' world: what is the ground of their isolation? Therapists can offer clients a relationship which confirms clients as competent social beings – e.g. a relationship in which there are clear yet flexible boundaries, an appropriate interchange of roles, an exploration of closeness-distance issues within the therapeutic relationship, an understanding of different perspectives, respect for the other and an awareness of disconfirming attitudes and behaviours.
Generativity/stagnation	Therapists can imagine the real of their clients' world: what underlies their stagnation? Therapists can explore with clients how they might provide a context for the future and prepare for the next generation – e.g. effective parenting and creative endeavours such as composing work schedules, commitments of non-abuse, certificates of reconciliation, etc. These tasks can invite clients to confirm themselves as productive beings.
Ego-integrity/despair	Therapists can imagine the real of their clients' world: what is the ground of their despair? Therapists can reflect with clients on past experiences, warming to remembered successes, and inviting clients' self-acceptance of past disappointments, missed opportunities and old regrets, finding ways for clients to confirm themselves as integrated beings.

Yet other contraries have been touched upon in the stories above. Bernadette has left single life to become a couple with Daniel whereas Jason is concluding marriage and making the transit to individual living. Bernadette is facing early mid-life issues whereas Jason's crises are those of late mid-life. Hence, Bernadette's options are expanding whereas Jason is looking back: gathering the loose, tangled threads and completing his tapestry; a tattered hole here, a muddy patch there but, as an entity, effectively woven and well hung. Finally, the paradox of creativity, explored by Frank Barron in his

Minnesota Multiphasic Personality Inventory (MMPI) researches on gifted students (Getzels 1962) appears relevant: that creative people appear more neurotic or psychotic on measures of anxiety, depression, schizophrenia and deviance but are paragons of stability on measures such as ego-strength (i.e. the power to rally from set-back). Stimulating Bernadette's and Jason's creative potentials appeared to help them bounce back, cope with their adversity and reconcile the contraries in their lives (Barron 1968).

The way people experience their world will depend on whether they assume an I–It or an I–Thou position. They will interpret and make meaning of their world according to whichever position is predominant. For those persons who constantly assume an I–It position, the world is filled with either people waiting to be used and exploited or people whose aim is to use and exploit others. For those who have entered an I–Thou position, the world is filled with others who are connected, who share a common experience, who are also willing to enter an I–Thou position to experience, explore and discover within relationship. People also designate qualities within themselves and in others according to these two positions. Those who assume an I–It position will often label themselves or others as either 'good' or 'bad', 'polite' or 'rebellious', 'kind' or 'cruel' or 'industrious' or 'lazy'. People who enter an I–Thou position will be able to detect both positive and negative qualities that are contrary to the actual 'good'/'bad' labels, that is both 'polite' and 'dull', 'rebellious' and 'innovative', 'kind' and 'patronizing', 'cruel' and 'disciplined', 'industrious' and obsessive', 'lazy' and 'carefree'. Whenever clients label themselves or their intimates as 'dull', 'rebellious' or 'obsessive', therapists can confirm the personhood of the blamed clients by highlighting the positive contrary quality: 'polite', 'innovative' or 'industrious'. When people converse and are willing to enter an I–Thou position with one another, they can start to *imagine the real* of each other's experience. *Imagining the real* is a term that Buber used to describe the process of entering 'into the life of the Other' (Buber 1965b, p.81) – a process in which all one's skills and resources are utilized to understand what the other is experiencing. This is an essential quality of therapy. The therapist must suspend all assumptions about the person(s) he or she is facing, listen clearly to the conversation and convey to the clients that they are being understood. By *imagining the real* of the clients and revealing that they have been heard, the therapist is participating in what Buber terms *inclusion*. *Inclusion* occurs when therapists *imagine the real* of their clients with such clarity that the therapists are able to regard both their own and their clients' beliefs as valid. Initially, it is the therapist who spends most energy *imagining the real* of the client. As therapy proceeds, with a willingness of clients to enter the I–Thou position, there occurs a mutual act of *inclusion*. Both therapist and client gain an understanding and appreciation of each other; both recognize each other as being participants included within the human drama.

Case 1F: a hidden message[9]
Lesley, 28 years, felt that she would never be able to control her daughter Marnie, aged 8. For weeks, Marnie had been throwing tantrums and hitting her stepsister Tessa, aged 3. Lesley had separated from Marnie's father four

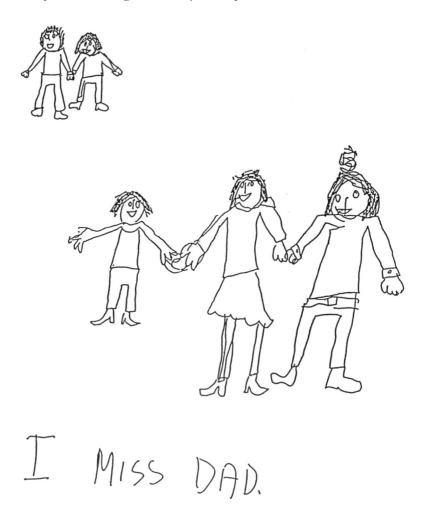

Figure 1.3 Marnie's drawing

9   This case was originally presented in *Patient Managment 14*, August 1990, 101–8.

years previously. As I talked with Lesley, I asked Marnie to draw picture of the family (see Figure 1.3). Marnie folded the paper t| her into two and drew, on the front page, a picture of the family – ,.. included her mother and father standing close together, holding hands. Lesley's new friend and Tessa (their offspring) were drawn as very small figures, placed in the background. As I chatted with Lesley about the picture (how her daughter still saw Lesley and her husband as a pair, with Tessa and her father not yet part of the family) Marnie interjected: 'You have not looked inside the book yet'. I opened the folded paper and read Marnie's words inside: 'I miss Dad'. Lesley and I discussed access arrangements. As it happened, Marnie had not seen her father for the previous eighteen months. I asked Marnie if she would ring her father and let him know that she missed him, that she wanted to see him; perhaps he did not know? Two months later, Marnie has telephoned and visited her father and the tantrums have ceased.

Discussion

Lesley can be regarded as viewing her parenting of Marnie within an I–It position. Lesley considered herself as an 'It', a 'bad mother' who was raising Marnie, also an 'It', a 'bad child'. To have offered parent-effectiveness training at this stage might well have increased Lesley's sense of self-blame and of being an 'It'. Instead, the therapist encouraged Marnie to draw her perception of the family and used the picture to include Lesley, Marnie and himself within another framework. Marnie's drawing communicated quite clearly the context of her distress: her isolation from her father. Including all participants within Marnie's perspective put the problem within a different context, from 'Lesley's ineffective parenting of an outrageous child' to 'Marnie's response to her parents' divorce, missing father and wishing that the former family was reconstituted'. The drawing made it easier for Lesley, Marnie and therapist to meet with each other within an I–Thou position and seek a different solution, one which also included Marnie's father. Marnie was enabled to gain some power over her life, approach her father and let him know her needs.

These concepts of *meeting* within an I–Thou position, *imagining the real*, and *inclusion* are all encompassed by a conversational space that Buber calls the *Between*. For Buber, 'the Between is not objective, not subjective, nor the sum of the two… (Wood 1969, p.41). It is a space in which 'the interhuman blossoms into genuine dialogue' (Buber 1965, p.81), where solutions evolve, clients exclaim 'I never thought of it like that before!', where the 'Aha!' occurs and magic happens.

Case 1G: Louella[10]

Louella, 30 years, was referred to me by her general practitioner because of her feelings of 'depression'. An only child, she had lost her mother to an illness when she was 14 years old. Although she had stayed with her father after her mother's death, Louella had come under the influence of her mother's sister. Both her mother and aunt were fundamentalist in their religious practices, stressing the evils of sexual relationships before and within marriage, the positive power of prayer, reward and the punishment of Hell eternal, and the importance of adhering to the 'right way'. Louella said that her mother had had to marry her father because she was pregnant at the time with her. The mother had also been conceived out of wedlock and was the reason for the grandparents' marriage. Louella said that she was always a 'good girl' during her teen years, always trying to make her aunt happy, and that she was shy of men generally. In spite of this, Louella had met Scott, with whom she had lived for six years and with whom she had given birth to Joseph, now aged two-and-a-half, born out of wedlock. Louella had parted with Scott eighteen months previously because 'he had relied so heavily on her to cater to his every need'. He had typecast Louella into the 'wife–mother' role and had not been prepared to share domestic responsibilities mutually or reliably. Louella's father had died five years previously.

The initial sessions of therapy, seeing Louella individually, were spent in doing grief work and exploring relationship problems within Louella's network. Two generations – mother and grandmother – appeared to have had difficulties integrating sexual and spiritual attitudes, and I wondered if this was not a theme in Louella's life-script.

I have been interested for many years in the use of cinema as a therapeutic medium, encouraging clients to see films and discuss whether the themes in the films apply to themes within the clients' lives. I have found cinema an invaluable tool to include clients and myself within the whole field of human interaction. In the film *Labyrinth*, the main character is Sarah, whose entrance into puberty is complicated by her parents' divorce, her father's re-marriage and the birth of her stepbrother. Sarah is left one evening to care for the toddler. In a fit of pique, she wishes him 'away with the goblins'. David Bowie, as the goblin king, is only too happy to oblige and Sarah must traverse the labyrinth to the goblin king's palace to rescue her ward. On the way, Sarah meets many strange creatures: Hoggle, the reluctant dwarf; the strong,

---

10 This case was originally presented in *Journal of Integrative and Eclectic Psychotherapy*, 8, 1, Spring 1989, 3–6.

but frightened, shaggy monster; the bird with two heads always competing with each other; the small, gallant and fearless fox; the old woman who hoards trash and offers every piece as treasure; and a flock of flamingos who are able to disengage parts of their bodies and encourage Sarah to take risks and do the same. All throughout the journey, the goblin king tempts Sarah: 'Stay with me and I will give you the world'. Sarah does make her way through the labyrinth, retrieves her stepbrother and, with the help of her friends, overcomes the goblin king and his minions. At the film's end, Sarah's friends are about to depart when Hoggle says: 'We don't have to leave, we can be with you whenever you wish', to which Sarah responds: 'Oh please don't go completely. I never want to lose you entirely'. And all the friends and Sarah have a wonderful celebration! To me, this film is a clever representation of the path through adolescence where many strange and bizarre experiences are encountered and need to be addressed. Erik Erikson (1968) claims that adolescents seek emancipation from parents, control of sexual and aggressive drives, an ability to abstract meaning for their lives and a secure and certain sense of self that remains no matter what the circumstance. In traversing the labyrinth, one may accept the goblin king's offer and dwell there as an aging adolescent, or re-integrate those experiences encountered and complete the journey into mature adulthood – a state, I guess, in which one can choose to be as adolescent as the context and ethics afford. Just as Sarah decided where and when to party with her friends, so might we select which adolescent qualities we might use to enhance our adult living, for example to fuel our creativity, exploration, innovation, curiosity and sense of fun.

I suggested that Louella view *Labyrinth* and, after she had done so, asked: 'What qualities do you remember of those people who most influenced you during your teen years?' Louella first mentioned Cynthia, a schoolmate who had impressed with her calm and stable demeanour. Another chum, Jenny, was gentle at times, and at others, zany and full of energy. Louella described her mother as 'distant and uncaring'. Louella had been always running away to her friends' homes to escape. Louella described her mother as nervous and a religious autocrat. Louella said that her teachers had taught her to question dogma and absolute truths and she had valued the opportunity to differ from her family's perspectives.

I continued: What if Louella were to arrange a celebration similar to that at the end of *Labyrinth*? Which qualities of those people would she invite along? Louella replied: 'A consistent level of calm and stability, a flexibility between softness and zany fun, and an ability to question the dilemmas of the world'. I commented that, in the film, some of Sarah's friends had not been altogether pleasant. They had been bizarre, and sometimes a bit scary, and it had taken a little lateral thinking to comprehend their usefulness. Perhaps her mother's anxiety might be considered a teaching tool, guiding Louella to be cautious when appropriate. 'Yes', replied Louella, catching the drift of our dialogue, 'her religious ways did give me some disciplines and her aloofness enabled me to be independent and reach out to my friends. (with tears) I think that she wanted me to achieve independence because she realized that she was dying and knew that I would have to spend a large part of my life without her presence'.

And so our conversation continued, affirming those parts of Louella's adolescent experience that nourished her, finding ways to re-frame those parts that she found irksome as useful within a different context, mutually defining concepts, behaviours and values that we shared or that were uniquely each of ours alone. Our encounter, which had commenced with client requesting help from therapist, concluded as an existential meeting of equals.

Buber described the conclusion of therapy as an existential meeting of equals as *confirmation*: 'the wish of every man to be confirmed as what he is, even as what he can become' and 'the innate capacity in man to confirm his fellow man in this way' (Buber 1965, pp.67ff; Friedman 1960, 1985, p.119). A successful therapy can be regarded as one that *confirms* both therapist and client as competent human beings, sometimes connected during the conversation, sometimes apart and respecting each other's privacy, free to challenge each other without disconfirming one another. Therapy ends when both therapist and client acknowledge one another as mutual participants within the human drama, available to contact each other or leave each other alone, at will.

> 'Once upon a time,' said Bunam, 'in a simple public house in Warsaw, I heard two Jewish potters at a neighboring table tell each other all kinds of things over their brandy. One of them asked: "Have you learned the Scripture portion for this week?" "Yes", said the other. "So have I," said the first one, "and I find one thing hard to understand. It says there concerning our father Abraham and Abimelech, the king of the Philistines: 'They made, these two, a covenant.' I asked myself why it says: 'These two.' That seemed superfluous." "A good question," cried the other. "But how do you answer that question?" "I think," the other answered, "they made a covenant, but they did not become one; they remained two."'

'Granted,' replied the Yehudi. 'But, be they Philistines, or servants of Abraham...how far shall we carry the distinction? Are only the latter to be redeemed and not the former too? When we say, "Redemption of the World", do we mean only the redemption of the good? Does not redemption primarily mean the redeeming of the evil from the evil ones that make it so? If the world is to be forevermore divided between God and Satan, how dare we say that it is God's world? You say: those two were not one. Granted. But is that to remain true to the very end of days? And if they are ultimately to become one, when will that becoming begin?' (Buber 1981, pp.120–1)

A personal reflection

My mother Eva Gunzburg, who met Buber, writes: One of Martin Buber's contributions not yet mentioned was his enormous influence on the German language through his translation of the Torah from the original Hebrew. All other translations, even the King James Bible, are from the Greek translation, the Septuagint (said to have been made by 72 Jewish scholars in 72 days at the request of Ptolemy II). Needless to say, Buber's influence on Jewish thinking was also tremendous. Martin Buber was only the second German to do such a translation, the first being the other Martin, namely Luther.

My 'friend' Martin called his book *die Funf Bucher der Weisung* – *the Five Books of Instruction*. His co-operator was Franz Rosenzweig, an eminent Jew and Hebraist, who lived in Frankfurt am Main (one of the greatest centres of Jewish culture in the 1920s) who unfortunately, like so many scholars, died before the book went to press. The two most cherished books in my library are Martin's *Funf Bucher (Vol 1)* and Franz Rosenzweig's *Briefe (Letters)*. They formed my schooling into Jewish awareness. I attended the final seminar that Martin Buber gave to us twenty-five youth leaders on the farm run by Schocken, his publisher. We were all preparing for our emigration, including Martin (or, in Hebrew, Mordechai) as he wanted to be called. I was, of course, Chavah (my Hebrew name). It was a weekend affair: Shabbat evening with songs past midnight, early Shabbat morning service, midday meal with all the trimmings, tutorials in the afternoon, etc. The three most memorable facts that came out of this occasion were:

1. The Shabbat evening meal consisted of fruit soup (it was mid-August, the hottest month in Europe), hot dogs and strawberries without cream. Hot dogs you ask?? Well, the beautiful breast of veal (specially slaughtered for this great occasion) was in the insides of the 'so called' farm watch-dog who had raided the

Coolgardie-type cooler during the night. As it was too late to get the slaughterer out from Berlin to prepare another calf, we all, including Martin, set out to kill chickens, pluck and cook them for Shabbat Day dinner and we put them into the padlocked Dutch Oven to cook. Martin taught us how to kill a chicken according to Jewish ritual. Martin gave us a whole lecture on food acceptable for a Shabbat meal. As you may know from his talks, the poor ate just potatoes during the week and added a herring to their festive fare.

2. At the first tutorial Martin gave us a 'puzzle' as he called it. Were each of us Jewish because our parents and grandparents were so? Did we go to Synagogue on Festivals (Saturday was a schoolday in state schools in Germany) because the family went and it was expected of us or did we go of our own volition and conviction? (By the way, the participants – five girls and twenty boys – were all in their early to mid-twenties and two couples were to marry before migration).

3. This was the most important and impressive. It was Martin's final and farewell address in which he urged everyone of us, whether we followed him to the Promised Land or were scattered to the corners of the globe, to carry ourselves proudly as Jews; to be steadfast and direct some of our leisure daily to some aspect of Jewishness, either in study, devotion, contemplation, or practices, and to be aware that we were not only Jews but Menschen and to act with humanity. 'Go forth', he said, 'and be my ambassadors!' He blessed us all with appropriate blessings, wished us all Shalom and L'Hitraot and drove off into the night on his journey to Israel.

Endnote

There is not room in this book for a comprehensive account of how the author structures the therapy in which he participates. For a greater understanding, readers are recommended to refer to Gunzburg (1993) Chapters 3 and 4 and Gunzburg and Stewart (1994) Chapters 2, 3, 4 and 5.

Section Two

Bibliotherapy: the art of book-healing

> The therapy of all therapies is not to attach oneself exclusively to any particular therapy, so that no illusion may survive of some end beyond an intensely private sense of well-being to be generated in the living of life itself. (Rieff 1968, p.261)

The power of story

Martin Buber believed in the potent healing effect of story on the aching soul. He understood story to be a medium within which various existential themes of life – belonging, yearning for companionship, loss of homeland, courage in adversity, the blossoming of love – could be woven and transmitted from one group to another and from one generation to the next. The telling of story could convey the struggle to understand the mystery of life, the dilemmas encountered and the myriad ways that such challenges could be met. Above all, story could convey both the uniqueness of individual experiencing and the connectedness of all living things.

William Stewart writes:

> Many therapists use the principles of what is known as 'Bibliotherapy'. The Greek meaning of Bibliotherapy is 'book-healing', the aim of which is to create a psychological interplay between the reader and the material, which may be literature or audio-visual.

> The relationship so formed may then be used to promote insight, personal awareness and growth and psychological healing. It achieves this through overcoming moralization, active involvement and fostering competence.

> Bibliotherapy is often used as an adjunct to other forms of therapy. It may be conducted in a one-to-one relationship or in a group. It is used with client groups of all ages. People be helped through a story, play, music, songs, to explore major themes of life which are creating difficulties for them.

> Bibliotherapy can be helpful with people who have emotional or behavioural problems, where the objective is insight or behavioural change. The empathic or imaginative nature of the material would aim to produce catharsis.
>
> It may also be used with people who, apart from passing through a crisis, are not psychiatrically disturbed. The goal is self-actualization and growth through using both imaginative and directive, factual material.
>
> The rationale is that people are encouraged to deal with their own threatening emotions and behaviours by displacing them on to the story. Identification takes place with the characters which promotes change. (Gunzburg and Stewart 1994, p.130–1)

Carmel Flaskas comments:

> There is a richness in the processes of counselling and therapy which often becomes lost in the translation to the case study format. The richness lies mainly in the life experiences of people who come for therapy, in the woven fabric of histories, in the pain of loss and abuse, and capacity of people to hope for something better and to struggle for something better. It is also very hard in casebook descriptions to capture a sense of the relationship between the therapist and clients and to present a particular process of therapy in all its specificity... (Gunzburg and Stewart 1994, pp.9–10)

Flaskas highlights some important points in the telling of stories:

- That descriptions of our work with clients be accessible, warm and honest and display the experience we have as therapists.

- That it is possible to write of therapy experiences in a way which does not reduce our clients' experiences or the therapy process itself.

- That in presenting our case work, we do not assume the privileged position of giving 'the truth' about our clients' experiences, or even about the therapy process itself; rather we give our own reflections on our clients' situations and the therapy work.

- That our stories provide a constant invitation for readers/listeners to engage with the clinical material and commentaries and to further reflect from their own positions.

- That our stories can offer a systematic discussion of the main issues, ethics and skills that are all part-and-parcel of therapeutic work.

- That our stories can convey ideas about therapeutic techniques and teach how to locate ourselves personally in our relationships with our clients.

- That our stories allow for the complexities and uncertainties of our clients' situations and maintain a clarity of therapeutic focus.

In Section Two, I want to present a series of case studies which illustrate how, in sharing the case studies with our clients, the clients can be invited to reflect on their own situation. I want to stimulate therapists to build up their own collection of case studies from their own experience so that they can enhance the quality of their therapeutic conversation. Through the telling of stories to clients, we can achieve some of Buber's conditions for an effective therapeutic conversation to which we referred in Section One:

- the need for therapists and clients to *meet*

- the need for therapists to *imagine the real* of their clients' experience so that therapists and clients together can be *included* within the therapeutic conversation

- the need for therapists and clients to be *confirmed* by the therapeutic conversation.

I hope to show how the sharing of stories can facilitate all these processes and lead to effective, enriched and rewarding therapy.

Mapping the therapeutic conversation

Buber did not consider that our experiences were grounded within abstract ideas or theoretical dogmas, yet so much of the conversation in which therapists participate is based on just that: ideas that have become frozen into structures and codes which prevent, rather than facilitate, the experiencing of the therapeutic process. Often, the founders of various schools of therapy displayed great brilliance and innovation in their original thought and activity and, as the schools which arose out of their philosophy developed, their concepts came to be regarded as 'holy writ'. The original 'Masters' had spoken and their early devotees created a body of sacred lore and ritual that all who came after were obliged to follow. More recently, with the advent of feminism and the acknowledgement of the oppression of women and indigenous populations, therapists have swung away from theories which attempt to offer universal explanations of human psychological functioning.

Rather, they have focused on the valuing of difference and prizing of diversity that is to be found between, and within, various social and cultural groups. The emphasis is more now on 'participating within counselling. We are more likely to engage our clients within narrative or conversation, to co-operate, co-create and hear different voices (Stagoll 1991), to pay attention to emotionality (Smith *et al.* 1990) and introduce issues of responsibility (Jenkins 1990), safety and social justice (Waldegrave 1990)' (Gunzburg and Stewart 1994, p.44).

And yet it is essential to have some guidelines and structure to therapy otherwise all may become chaos and amorphous, a conversation that winds round and round, a never-ending story. When considering how to conduct a therapeutic conversation and which story to share with clients, it is useful to keep in mind a number of ideas from the various theories that abound and to remember that these ideas are not absolute rules for conducting therapy. Rather, the ideas can represent conceptual 'maps', tools to help gather and organize information, and to construct our stories during the therapeutic encounter. Buber would stress that *our* maps are not the territory and that the way we therapists view what is happening will change as therapy proceeds and we reflect on our experiences during our conversational journey. The value of having a number of maps in mind is that they can help us link into the maps that our clients are using to make sense of their world. Thus we can imagine their reality, enter it and meet them on their own ground. Also pertinent is that the maps offered below were largely formulated within western culture and that very different perspectives and stories may be necessary when conversing with clients from diverse ethnic origins. The process of presentation of these maps is as follows: a single concept from each map which I have found useful in conversing with clients is offered and then a story follows, illustrating how I convey that idea to clients. The usefulness of conveying an idea in this manner is that it can open up a different avenue of inquiry to clients. For a client who is overwhelmed with self-blame, and constantly searching for a cure for some perceived defect within, a story conveying an idea from the systemic map, indicating that there are many complex factors within the client's family and society that may be contributing to his or her woes, can create significant impact. On the other hand, I would invite a man who is abusing his female partner and blaming her for her perceived domestic incompetence to consider some ideas from the feminist map: how do men learn to violate partners whom they profess to love? What would it be like to have a partner who loved and respected him rather than related towards him in fear?

Finally, there is a discussion section following each case study in which I try to reveal to the reader my understanding of what I was experiencing throughout the therapeutic conversation and what was the effector of change. The actual case descriptions are my understanding of what was happening during the therapy at the time, whereas the discussion sections are my way of stepping back from the therapeutic meeting and reflecting on it. As Carmel Flaskas (Gunzburg and Stewart 1994), puts it:

> In presenting his casework, John does not assume the privileged position of giving 'the truth' about his clients' experiences, or even about the therapy process itself. Rather, he gives his own reflections on his clients' situations and the therapy work...so that...there is a constant invitation for readers to engage with the clinical material and commentaries and to further reflect from their own positions on the counselling issues... (pp.9–10)

These, of course, are only my ideas and fancies and I take full responsibility for the flaws, biases and prejudices contained in them. Another therapist might have quite different ways of explaining the material presented. If readers are stimulated to reflect on how these cases differ from their own work, and that reflection proves to generate new ideas and new ways of participating in therapy for them, I will consider the whole venture to have been successful.

I also wondered whether to change some of the syntax and phraseology in which I had written the earlier casework from the 80s. Although I no longer use some of those descriptions, I have decided to keep the descriptions as I wrote them. Readers will be able to compare those earlier case descriptions with cases written in the 90s, to examine the process of development of therapeutic practice over several years. Throughout, Buber's ideas are included to illustrate how they can nourish therapy, no matter what therapeutic map is being used.

A cautionary note

Readers will have noted from the case studies presented that I am very self-revealing during the therapy in which I participate. I find that, at particular moments, sharing self-experience can increase the client's options for their own self-exploration – as in the case of sharing a drawing with Bess (Case 1C, p.9), a professional paper with Bernadette (Case 1D, p.12) and my passionate interest in film as a therapeutic medium with Louella (Case 1G, p.22). The purpose of self-revelation is to facilitate meeting between therapist and client; to share the common humanity of the struggle. The danger of self-revelation is that it can be delivered in a patronizing and self-serving manner, that is the therapist says: 'Oh, I know what you are talking about! This situation happened to me too. This is what I did. Why don't you try this too?' Such a message can leave the client discomforted, thinking: 'Oh isn't he/she clever? Why couldn't I be clever like that too?' A more useful message behind the self-revelation is for the therapist to offer: 'A similar thing happened to me. This was part of my story too…and I guess I am telling you my story because this issue of (say, belonging, patriarchal oppression, loss) influences both our stories. What are some of the ways that you could rewrite your story?' As a therapist, I do not share my solutions to the struggle with my clients. I emphasize that we are here to search for their options, not mine. It is absolutely essential that self-revelation is not undertaken in isolation, that is that therapists have a professional network of peers with whom they can discuss their casework and receive supervision regularly. At times it may be necessary to seek psychotherapy. Our clients can trigger off all sorts of unexpected reactions, particularly if they are violent to self or other. Currently, my supportive network is family, friends and colleagues. I have had some years of psychotherapy in the past,though not for the last ten years.

Yet this is my dilemma. With all my self-exploration and self-knowledge, I am never certain how I know when to reveal some aspect of my own experience to a client. I must not be self-revealing to the client's detriment. I must pace the client's conversation and listen carefully to his or her needs at any given moment. But moments of intimacy and entering an I–Thou position is not willed. It is during such moments, when I and my client are most connected, that I have found self-revealing will often open up a new area for the client to explore. I can never be sure. I can only keep participating in therapy, keep talking to my colleagues, keep writing and keep reflecting.

Setting the scene: encouraging meeting

Martin Buber's concept of *meeting* very much resembles Donald Winnicott's notion of the *holding environment* or *facilitating environment*. This idea, which forms the basis for therapist and client engaging one another, refers to the conditions of security and hope that a parent offers a child and, analogously, that a therapist furnishes a client (Winnicott 1965). Leupnitz (1988) comments that every kind of therapy has some version of the *holding environment*. For instance, Freud (1960) used the metaphor of 'breast-feeding' that occurred between therapist and client when psychoanalysis was proceeding effectively. Laing (1965) regarded adequate therapy as being an authentic meeting of 'true selves' and Rogers (1975) considered therapy to be proceeding well when therapists were 'congruent' with their clients; they were meeting within an atmosphere of warmth, empathy and unconditional acceptance. Maslow (1968) talked of the therapeutic encounter as providing a basic level where clients' safety needs were satisfied and Erikson (1968) postulated that a therapeutic environment had to be established so that clients would experience the 'basic trust' that, perhaps, they had not developed during their infancy.

Winnicott also introduced the phrase *good-enough mothering* indicating that effective parenting did not necessitate perfect child-rearing practices but rather, adequate nurturing and guidance. Similarly, *meeting* between therapist and client can be regarded as not depending on absolute theoretical dogmas or expert techniques but rather, on a sufficiently informed conversation within a *holding environment* by a *good-enough therapist*.[1]

Case 2A: Mum loves me

June, 1990: Norton, 11 years, was telling me about his life at school. A likeable lad, with blue eyes and blonde hair cut with a wisp down the back of his neck as was the current fashion, Norton had proven to be one of the most popular boys at his school. He had many friends, was dedicated to his studies and was an enthusiastic participant in cricket and football. His only problem, as he told it, was that sometimes he would occasionally get a bit 'down in the dumps' and would throw tantrums and become embroiled with his mother, Maureen, 27 years.

Frankly, I was surprised that Norton was not more delinquent in his behaviour. His father Jim, 29 years, a bricklayer, had disappeared when Norton was three. Maureen, a survivor of childhood sexual abuse, was unemployed and relied on alcohol for succour. Norton could not remember Maureen ever having been sober for more than a couple of days' duration. Maureen's boyfriend Trent, 25 years, a printer, was still troubled by the effects of his father's physical abuse during childhood. In fact, Trent had been seeing me in therapy for some months – to get a handle on his rage and own alcohol abuse – and Norton was very much a 'visitor', attending our session to meet Trent's 'therapeutic friend'.

I complimented Norton on his academic, social and sporting successes. I thought it remarkable that, with Maureen and Trent having such a struggle with their drinking problems, Norton was able to do so well. I commented

---

1   This section, including Cases 2A and 2B, is based on an article that was originally presented in the 'General Practitioner' *Adis International 1*, 4, April 1993, 9.

that kids from such families would often get angry and be violent, would steal, or be depressed, or use drugs and drink alcohol to excess themselves. How had Norton found the strength and ability to overcome these struggles within his family? 'Oh, I'm all right', Norton responded immediately, "cos Mum loves me'. I had not heard a youth so certain of his mother's love before. So many people seek therapy with me because they experience a lack of parental love. 'It's great that your Mum loves you', I said, 'How can you be so sure?'. 'Because', Norton replied, 'when she was pregnant with me, she said that she gave up drinking and smoking for the whole time she was carrying me. She said that she was going to be darned sure that I was not going to be born abnormal'.

Case 2B: A bowl of soup

November, 1992: Shirley, 39 years, a cashier, was distressed, depressed and berating God yet again. 'Why doesn't He listen to me?', she mourned, 'I keep asking Him to make my life just a little better. I am a good Jewish girl. Why...doesn't... He... HEAR me!?!'.

Shirley and her husband Joe, 47 years, a taxi-driver, had made few financial gains over the past twenty years of their marriage and were particularly stretched due to the economic recession of 1992. 'I only clear two hundred dollars a week', Shirley continued, 'Joe brings home about the same. What can we do with four hundred dollars a week?' 'Listen', I responded, 'would you save two dollars a week and, every fortnight, go to Singer's Good Food Eating Company and treat yourself to a bowl of soup. For that price you also get thrown in a couple of delicious pieces of wholemeal bread. If you are slowly going under, two dollars a week spent on yourself is not going to be missed'. 'Thank you, God!', Shirley snorted, 'A bowl of soup...thank you very much indeed!'. 'Is that what it is all about then?', I queried, 'Is that why God is not tossing the big stuff your way? I imagine He does not waste his gifts. If you don't appreciate the small things, is that why he is overlooking you for first prize?' 'Oh', said Shirley, ceasing her tirade.

By our next weekly session her spirits had lifted and both she and Joe had supped on Singer's soup. Six months later, Joe had received permanent employment as a bus-driver with livable hours and improved pay!

Discussion

Both these cases illustrate the application of *meeting* through *good-enough mothering*. Maureen, despite her human foibles, was able to transmit to Norton a message that she loved him enough to ensure that he would not be deformed during pregnancy by her abstaining from drinking and smoking. Shirley was able to change her view of God from an unforgiving, unrewarding, punitive Deity to one who might give small gifts regularly. This is not to be confused with a flippant 'count your blessings and be thankful for what you have!' approach. Rather, the questions invited of Shirley were: Does God deal in small gifts? Are these gifts adequate for physical, emotional and spiritual sustenance? Indeed, is God a *good-enough mother*? Does receiving these small gifts offer hope? Having regained hope, does this create a mental set to recognise larger gifts as they are offered?'

Therapists can encourage the process of *meeting* between themselves and their clients by being empathic – by sensing and non-judgmentally reflecting their feelings and meanings. As Carl Rogers (1980) says:

> Rarely do we listen with real understanding, true empathy, yet listening, of this very special kind, is one of the most potent forces for change that I know. Three conditions during therapy – genuineness, acceptance and empathy – are the water, the sun, and the nutrients that enable survivors of abuse to grow like strong, vigorous oak trees. As persons are accepted and prized, they tend to develop a more caring attitude toward themselves. As persons are empathically heard, it becomes possible for them to listen more accurately to the flow of inner experiencings (p.116).

When therapists drop their façades and express genuinely their true feelings, when they enable their clients to feel unconditionally accepted, and when they sense and reflect their clients' feelings empathically, the clients may grow in their self-understanding and self-acceptance. To paraphrase Rogers (1980, p.10): Therapists hearing their clients has consequences. When a therapist truly hears clients and the meanings that are important to them at that moment, hearing not simply their words, but them, and when the therapist lets them know that their own private personal meanings have been heard, many things can happen. There may first of all be a grateful look, they may feel released, they may want to tell the therapist more about their world, they may surge forth in a new sense of freedom to they may become more open to the process of change. The more deeply does the therapist hear their meanings, the more there may be that happens. Almost always, when people realize that they have been heard, their eyes moisten. It is as though they were saying 'Thank God, somebody heard me. Someone knows what it is like to be me'.

Speaking the client's language

It can be helpful in establishing and maintaining *meeting* for therapists to match their phraseology, metaphors, voice tones and energy levels with those of their clients. Norton was a bright young lad and so I spoke to him in a lively, practical patter that did not contain too many long sentences. The films that we discussed included *Boyz n'the Hood* and *Jurassic Park* – both dealing with survival against hostile forces. With Shirley, the mood of conversation was slower and the vocabulary more eloquent, verging almost on the lyrical. We talked about films such as *Enchanted April* and *Sleepless in Seattle* – both to do with finding almost magical solutions to heartaches. In the case study below, I was able to find a link between my knowledge of music and the client's indigenous language that enabled us both to connect.

Case 2C: The solicitor[2]

December, 1992: Mahmoud, 44 years, a solicitor and refugee from Ethiopia, had come to Australia two years previously. He had suffered quite extraordinarily during the war in Africa, having been kept hostage by rebel forces for several months and being threatened with execution, before being rescued through the auspices of a medical colleague. Mahmoud's current dilemma was with his girlfriend Jessie, 36 years, a Melbourne-born welfare worker. They had known each other for about a year. Mahmoud said that he was very fond of Jessie and had considered a long-term partnership, yet Jessie was 'running hot and cold' and did not seem to know whether to commit herself to a future with Mahmoud or not. Some months ago, Jessie, originally from a Christian background and now an avowed atheist, had wanted to live with Mahmoud. This, however, had gone against the nature of Mahmoud's Islamic culture – marriage being the preferred option. Jessie had been married once before to Maurice, 44 years, a Jamaican architect who had abused alcohol and had physically violated her. Jessie's father had also misused alcohol and had beaten her throughout her youth. Though Mahmoud adhered to many of the ethical tenets of his faith, he said that he was not a fundamentalist and enjoyed the occasional social glass of wine. Whenever Jessie watched Mahmoud drink alcohol, she said that she was reminded of both her father's and ex-husband's abusive behaviour and became frightened. Mahmoud felt that perhaps his dark complexion reminded Jessie of Maurice. The issue had reached crisis point because Mahmoud was soon to sit for examinations that would enable him to practice

---

2   This case was originally presented in the 'General Practitioner', *Adis International 2*, 6, April 1994, 16.

as a barrister in Australia and he required a life-style with much less tension to study successfully.

I felt myself to be in a predicament also. How could I, as an Australian-born Jewish therapist from Russian/ Polish/ German ancestry and, having been trained initially as a general practitioner (often perceived as lower in the professional hierarchy than are solicitors/barristers), engage him within therapy?

Then I recalled that my father knew some Arabic. I remembered observing, as a lad, the beautiful script of his handwriting and listening to his mellifluous intonation as he recited verses from Arabic literature. I was a violinist. So I commenced discussing with Mahmoud my attraction to the musical patterns that I had noted within the Arabic language and compared them to the liquid tones of my stringed instrument. Mahmoud smiled...and relaxed more easily in his chair. He told me that he spoke five tongues. I mentioned that, besides English, my father spoke Hebrew and Russian well, a little Italian and French, with a smattering of Chinese. He loved to chase the root of a Hebrew word and trace it back to its origins. I mentioned my fondness for dialogue and narrative; how I would pursue a theme that arose during the therapeutic conversation and 'banter' it back and forth until it was clearly defined and sometimes redefined. It was rather like a stream of music with its harmonies and dissonances, crescendos and pauses, coda and finale. Mahmoud said that Jessie had commenced her own individual therapy a couple of weeks before with a female therapist. I suggested to Mahmoud that perhaps the most significant matter at hand was that he focus on passing his examinations. He had come to Melbourne to seek a better life after enduring horrific wartime abuses. Obtaining qualifications to practice a career within his expertise was important. Would he discuss with Jessie about creating a comfortable distance until his examinations were completed? During this time, she would be exploring her own development and Mahmoud would be concentrating on himself. After this time, they might then consider the pros and cons for reconciliation.

Mahmoud left my office and immediately made several weekly appointments to see me in the future.

Discussion

Mahmoud's quandary appeared to be whether to secure his career opportunities or pursue a relationship with Jessie. He had survived the ravages of war in Ethiopia and now wished to improve his lot in his new country. My predicament was how to invite Mahmoud, who came from a very different culture to mine, into therapy. I increased our sense of *meeting* by highlighting and affirming the similarities that we did share within my musical and Mahmoud's linguistic spheres, and suggested that the language of therapy imitates the flow of music. Our conversation appeared to put Mahmoud at ease and gave him permission to concentrate on his own needs for the moment: negotiating distance with Jessie to complete his studies.

Often clients will throw us a hook onto which we can hang and be drawn into their world, thus increasing the meeting between us, as the last case study illustrates.

Case 2D: The banquet manager
January, 1993: Carmel, 32 years, a banquet manager at a well-known hotel for some years, was describing her distress and anger at the manner in which her new boss Derek, 48, was discounting her, favouring two other male employees, who were younger and subordinate to her, over her. Carmel had found a caterpillar in a salad that one of the employees had made and, when she had disciplined the worker involved, Derek had 'tut-tutted' the whole matter, saying that she was making too much fuss over a minor event. Carmel's reputation up to that point had been flawless. Carmel believed that Derek was trying to get her to resign so that one of the other men would assume her position. She also felt that part of the problem was that Derek's wife had recently left him and that he was now abusing Carmel because she also was a woman. Carmel experienced herself as immobilized, not knowing which direction to take.

Carmel told a story of significant bereavement throughout much of her life. A twin sister had died two days after their birth and a friend, David, three years Carmel's senior, had been killed in a motor vehicle accident five years previously. Carmel and David had been planning a future together. I suggested that Carmel view the film *An Angel at my Table*, which depicts how Janet Frame, the New Zealand author, coped with similar losses.

'David should not have died on me', Carmel asserted at our next weekly meeting, after seeing the film. Carmel had warmed to the scene in which Janet Frame had enjoyed an intimacy with an American professor whilst visiting Spain. This moment had brought back many fond memories of her friendship with David. Carmel also described her horror at how a predominantly male medical profession had mistreated the author during her grief for two deceased sisters – a twin who had died at birth, another who had drowned in adolescence. The doctors had determined to perform lobotomy on her, only to change their decision when they learnt that she had won a literary award during the week before the proposed operation. 'I know that David's soul has gone to a better place but we could have had such a great life together if he had willed himself to live!', she said. 'So you believe in immortality, and spiritual continuity?', I queried. 'Yes', replied Carmel, 'I am not sure where David's soul has gone but I am sure he is well cared for wherever he is'. 'So in what part of the body do you believe the soul resides during life?', I continued. We discussed some of the traditional places that the soul has been thought to dwell: in the heart and in the pineal gland. 'You know', I said, 'I sometimes imagine that the soul might lie in the grey matter of the brain, within the cerebral cortex, because so much of our spiritual refreshment seems to be intimately connected with thinking. I wonder if that was David's problem? He was lying comatose for months in a hospital bed with a head injury before he died. There could not have been much of his cerebral cortex left alive. I wonder if his soul, being denied thinking processes and refreshment, was languishing and decided to seek spiritual nourishment elsewhere?' Carmel smiled... 'I like it', she said. 'You can have it', I replied.

Three months later Carmel has been dismissed by Derek and her position has been taken over by one of her former male staff. She has found new employment. She has written and posted a letter to Derek expressing clearly her feelings about his, and the other workers', violations. A female employee who remained at the hotel has recently told Carmel that she herself has been subject to humiliations from Derek and now fears for her job also.

Discussion

Carmel appeared to be overwhelmed in the face of death and emotional abuse from the men at work. We discussed whether Derek's behaviour towards her was misogynistic. A film was used to illustrate another woman's courageous struggles in overcoming comparable harsh odds. Carmel expressed her sense of desolation at her boyfriend's death some years earlier. She signaled her belief in the spiritual as a resource and in discussing how David's soul may have left his damaged body to seek comfort elsewhere, we increased our sense of *meeting*. This conversation seemed to offer Carmel consolation and renewed strength. After dismissal from her job, she obtained new employment and repudiated the abuse of her former colleagues in writing.

The systemic map

When clients enter my room blaming themselves for some hidden blemish or deficiency within and expecting me to join them in a lengthy search to uncover their hidden weakness, I encourage them to contemplate the idea that we can all be regarded as interconnected within one family system. Family members dance together in a complexity of harmonies which sometimes can create resounding discords. Often a member of a family can see himself at fault, whereas it is the interaction of family members with each other that can cause a person's internal discomfort. Moreover, there are many influences within the wider social system – economic pressures, cultural differences, patriarchal influences – which can lead to a person's experience of pain and unhappiness.

Case 2E: The journalist[3]

During her first therapy session, in October 1990, Claudine, 25 years, trained as a journalist but currently working in a clerical position, told me of the stress that had troubled her for months. She had experienced recurrent headaches, neck tension, insomnia and periods of disorientation and confusion. At times she had heard 'voices and vibrations' emanating towards her from pictures on the wall. Indeed, Claudine believed at times as if she was 'going crazy'. A psychiatrist had placed her on an anti-schizophrenic medicine. This had helped for a while, but now her voices were returning.

Claudine felt that part of her problem was work-related: the mother of Claudine's boss was dying of cancer and the boss appeared to be dumping the resentment and frustration caused by the mother's disability onto Claudine. Another problem was with Claudine's boyfriend, Len, 36 years, a theatre director, who said that he loved Claudine and planned a future with her but had made no plans to leave his other long-term lover. The actions of Claudine's boss and boyfriend seemed very much to replicate the patterns of abusive behaviour which Claudine's father, Abe, 53 years, unemployed for decades, had displayed towards her for as long as she could remember. Claudine was an only daughter. She described Abe as an 'anxious, depressed' man with a continuous history of psychiatric care and hospitalization. It sounded as if Abe had experienced no affection towards Claudine or her mother, Fay, 50 years, a clothing retailer, but rather was aggressively perfectionistic, demanding that Claudine achieve the most unreasonable academic standards. Abe himself had never been able to meet his own expectations and appeared to regard himself as something of a failure. Fay had been the power source and organizer of the family and Claudine felt that her mother was content in her lot and accepting of Abe's situation. Claudine remembered having been constantly frightened of Abe's temper outbursts during her adolescence.

---

3   This case was originally presented in *Psychotherapy in Australia 1*, 2, February 1995, 35.

Over our next several weekly meetings, I tried to build up a therapeutic atmosphere of safety and comfort for Claudine. I said that I admired Claudine's tenacity to survive such scary experiences with her father and commented that there would have been little time for fun or family content-ment. I wondered if Claudine was grieving over the missed opportunities for family closeness. It seemed to me that Abe had behaved like the typical patriarch, ordering everyone else around at his whim. Such abusive behaviour often caused severe stress and sometimes survivors were left wondering whether they were going mad or not.

I asked Claudine that if her internal emotional state could be described like a 'geographical territory' (Gunzburg 1991), what would hers be like? Claudine shared her description with me a week later:

> My land is an island. It is overwhelmingly barren and desolate. Many plants have tried to survive on this island but they inevitably wither and die in the scorching sun. The island is surrounded by sea but fresh water is scarce. Like all arid regions, this harbours its springs as a well-kept secret: buried unless interested explorers tap their sources. Limestone caves littered with old bones edge the beaches.

> Paradoxically, there are hidden pockets of lush forest which are dense and inaccessible. These are teeming with all sorts of wildlife, particularly the Snake and the Jaguar – untouched, wild and predatory.

> The island is easily accessible to neighbouring lands but it is not considered an appealing destination. It is more difficult to navigate the route from further afield.

Claudine's essay led to a discussion of what resources on the island may have been overlooked in despair at the isolation of the place. At a subsequent session, Claudine mentioned a group of melons growing at the border of the lush forest and that, in some nearby sand-dunes, some camels were wandering peacefully. Claudine felt that she might be able to tame one of the beasts and ride it to the melon patch to obtain nourishment. Our conversation gave rise to the theme of 'recognizing self-needs and having them met'. Abe seemed to have demanded his patriarchal rights from Claudine and her mother and did not appear to have acknowledged their wants. Out of this dialogue, Claudine was able to compose a series of assertive dialogues with Abe, encouraging him to acknowledge her more effectively.

Therapy lasted eight months – at the end of which, Claudine's symptoms had disappeared. She had resigned from working for her abusive boss and obtained a new position as editor of a society magazine. She had ended the friendship with Len and Abe too appeared to be well-distanced. Two years later, Claudine is married and remains symptom-free.

Discussion

Claudine described clearly the bodily symptoms and periods of bewilderment that signalled her distress. She related her problems to the behaviour of her boss and boyfriend but wondered if the fault was within her and if she was developing insanity. Because of Claudine's level of stress and to facilitate *meeting*, I decided to take things slowly and let Claudine develop her story at her own pace. *Imagining* Claudine's very real fear of 'impending madness', I encouraged Claudine to talk of her father Abe's autocratic and frightening behaviour throughout her childhood and of her mother's preoccupation with work and caring for the family and her invalid husband. Neither parent seemed to have had much time to nurture Claudine. She may have developed a sense of 'helplessness' which disempowered her now in adulthood, rendering her incapable of asserting herself to Abe and her abusive boss. The therapist *confirms* Claudine as having come through a difficult childhood and asked her to write an essay describing her internal 'emotional territory'. Through writing her essay, Claudine was able to 'name' her emptiness and desolation – resulting from Abe's discounts and the lack of parental nurturing – in her description of a deserted island.

This led the way to discussion of how Abe's abusive patriarchal behaviour might be the ground of Claudine's current distress, not some evolving mental illness, and that the violations of her boss and boyfriend may also be triggering off the memories of Abe's childhood abuse and so overwhelming Claudine. We considered how a patriarchal society created 'mad' women, slotting them into subservient roles in relation to men, and at the sacrifice of their own satisfaction. Were women condemned to work hard for their invalid men, support their distressed bosses and stand by patiently for their boyfriends to make important decisions? Such questions *confirmed* Claudine's ability to contest abuse. We were able to proceed towards conversation as to how Claudine might find nourishment on her island and she explored the metaphor further, finding ways to procure food. We talked about the importance of 'being heard and getting one's needs met' and Claudine then wrote some conversations in which she requested recognition of her needs as an independent adult from Abe. These further *confirmed* Claudine as a person who could protect herself practically from the abusers within her life, farewelling her boss and Len and creating distance with Abe.

Case 2F: The engineering student

March, 1992: Brko, 22 years, a fourth year electrical engineering student, described the episodes of internal fury that had threatened to break through his usually calm façade, and which had plagued him since childhood. Brko's father, Slobodan, who had died nine years previously from 'alcoholic cirrhosis', had constantly battered both Brko and his mother, Krystina, 52 years, and had sexually abused his sister Josie, 27 years. A year prior to his death, Slobodan had separated from Krystina. Two years later, Krystina had married Giuseppe, 52 years, a 'kind and decent man' who had given Brko a great deal of support. Brko could not understand then why now he should be so enraged. Slobodan was long dead and Krystina had found contentment. I expressed to Brko that, rather than finding him 'somehow deficient' in his current struggles, I was admiring of the way that he had endured his father's torment so well and presented himself now as a courteous young man wanting to discover a fairer way to life. At his next weekly session, Brko showed me a letter that I had invited him to write to Slobodan's 'ghost', contesting the abuse:

> Dear father,
>
> Why did you choose to leave your wife and children to fend for themselves in inevitable financial and emotional strain. Was the grog so powerfully mind-numbing to blind your sight of the love your family had for you or was it the selfishness you had for your own feelings that made you a prisoner of your own problematic world?
>
> There was never a time I can recall that my sister and I could please you with what we did. Yet other parents would reward their offspring for their efforts, we would only receive a nemesis. You would tell your friends how great we were at our academic level. Were the feelings of your friends more important than ours? We were never allowed to do exactly what we wanted or to be around friends we liked. Only the people you chose for us to be with.
>
> Yet at school I would excel in painting and writing and would win awards accrediting me of my natural ability but this was never exploited by you.
>
> We've come to terms with our grief and because of our love for God we are projecting ourselves to the goals we have all set ourselves. That goal is happiness.

Over our next three subsequent meetings, we discussed why Slobodan might have behaved in such a tyrannical manner. I introduced the theme of 'patriarchal privileges' and the idea that some men have that the world is made for them and that women and minors are there to serve their requirements. Brko gave up smoking 25 cigarettes per day and listed ten pieces of music that increased his internal sense of integration, including

Pachabel's 'Canon', Vivaldi's 'Four Seasons', Beethoven's 'Pastorale' symphony, J. S. Bach's 'Brandenburg' concertos and Mendelssohn's 'Italian' symphony. I was admiring that Brko was channelling the energy behind his anger into creative and health-giving activities and asked him what had made the difference. Brko replied: 'It was when I wrote my letter. It made me realize that we had loved my father and he had not responded in any way to our love'. I commented that often it was difficult for young men to develop their male identity when their fathers had abused them and I wondered if there was any positive quality that Slobodan might have bequeathed to him. Brko replied: 'He was a TV technician. I am sure that I got my love of electronics from him'. 'So, although your father's abuse was absolutely wrong, he was not a totally evil man?', I suggested, to which Brko smiled. Therapy lasted five weekly sessions. Six months later, Brko maintains his cool.

Discussion

Brko told of the internal anger that had been raging away beneath his calm exterior since childhood. As with Claudine, Brko blamed himself for an internal deficit that resulted in him feeling that way. This included the idea that he 'should' be happy in his life now that his abusive father was dead and buried and that his mother had entered a more rewarding relationship. The therapist wondered to himself if Brko was struggling with his own identity? Slobodan had provided Brko such an abusive image of manhood on which to model, I wondered how much of Brko's anger was grief at missed enjoyment within the family due to Slobodan's abuse? How much was self-hatred at his own masculinity? How much was frustration at his inability to change and become more contented? In order to *meet* Brko, I offered a more gentle model of manhood – one that invited Brko into conversation rather than one which demanded quick answers from him. Having *confirmed* Brko as a man concerned to seek equity in the future, so unlike his father, I encouraged him to write a letter to Slobodan's spirit – who still appeared to haunt him. In his letter, Brko 'names' Slobodan as a selfish, critical abuser who was unappreciative of, and rejected, the love of his family. Conversation moved toward a discussion with Brko that Slobodan had appeared to behave like 'the Master' in his home, demanding everybody else's attention at the expense of their own necessities. I invited Brko to re-examine his view that he 'should be alright now that Slobodan is dead', rather suggesting that the effects of abuse can run deep for many years after the events have stopped. Finally, we considered that, in composing his letter, Brko realised that there was genuine love for Slobodan within the family which his father had both discounted and violated. Brko had surely contested his father's abuse and *confirmed* himself as a man who could love both God and people! Brko had nominated music as a resource in his first session and I asked him to list a range of musical pieces that he found to be emotionally stabilizing. He also decided to quit smoking. I then asked if there is any gift that Slobodan might have bequeathed his son and Brko mentioned both men's fascination with electronics. It can difficult for a young man to define his masculinity when his father is an abuser. I have found it helpful to encourage survivors of abuse in identifying one or two positive qualities that they have chosen to take from abusers of the same gender. They then seem to be a little more assured in the development of their identity.

I read these stories to clients when I want to illustrate that therapy is very much an active venture in which both therapists and clients participate. There is a therapeutic meeting and conversation, then a break during which clients explore their world through experimental tasks. I mention that, during the break, therapists reflect on what has been spoken and usually converse with colleagues about the case; therapists are also explorers in this venture. Then there is a fresh encounter to reflect on the outcomes of the experiments and the therapists' thoughts and, together, to plot a future direction towards the next session.

The structural map

A well-functioning family can be considered as having a strong marital bond, clearly defined sub-systems and an effective parent-child hierarchy. Sub-systems can be regarded as having their own specific functions to nurture the psychosocial growth of individuals within them (Minuchin 1974). The marital sub-system, for example, would provide adult gratification and intimacy, self-growth and protection against stresses from the children. The sibling sub-system provides development of individual skills such as sharing, negotiating and co-operating, and the parental sub-system offers education, nurturing, guidance and discipline of the children. Pain in the family can occur when the marital bond is strained or when a child might enter an alliance with one parent against another. Therapy aims to re-balance the family so that the sub-systems can function effectively. Note that this description most adequately describes a 'traditional' husband-wife-children family and that a different map would be more appropriate with different family models, that is homosexual, communal, blended and single parent families.

Case 2G: Music to her ears[4]

January, 1992: Sonja, 31 years, a gardener, came to me after her previous therapist of nine years had died from a heart attack. Sonja felt that she had indeed killed him off, poisoning him with her evil nature.

As it happened, great evils had been perpetrated on Sonja during her childhood, including sexual abuse from her father, William – who had died from a heart attack six years previously – lack of protection and complete denial of the abuse from her mother, Elspeth, 62 years, and discounting and negativity by most members within her extended family. She had indeed been poisoned! For the first six months of weekly therapy, Sonja came to sessions dressed in shirts with sleeves rolled up, jeans and big hobnailed boots, with her hair tied tightly behind her head. Her message to me seemed to be quite clear: 'Get too close to me, buster, and I will stomp all over you!'

We talked about Sonja's obsession regarding knives. She would experience murderous thoughts towards all her friends and lovers, and had carefully locked away all knives in her kitchen. Sonja was terrified that one day she would stab a companion to death. Yet, behind her tough façade, Sonja occasionally let me glimpse brief flashes of a warm, tender and fun-loving interior. About six months into therapy, I commented: 'I hope one day you will let me see your soft, sensitive side'. Sonja shuddered visibly. Another six months passed, during which we discussed the nature of relationships: negotiating, sharing, arranging closeness-distance and the fair handling of power. Sonja agreed to collect all the knives that she did not need (enormous butcher's knives and all!) and put them in the dustbin on collection night. This she did. I also placed a fairly blunt letter-opener on the chair next to her in my room and, every few weeks, replaced it with a sharper blade, in an attempt to desensitize Sonja to the fear of her using it lethally.

Eventually, Sonja and I participated together in the ritual burning of a family photograph: the family that had participated in the sham of her 'happy childhood'. She scattered the ashes to sea off the local pier. This act seemed to create impact. About six weeks later, suddenly, out of the blue, Sonja attended our session dressed in a pastel multicoloured blouse and lilac skirt, with her hair hung down in long flowing tresses, and wearing lipstick. I felt touched and privileged, and said: 'Sonja, today you have given me a gift, something very special, a treasure that you do not easily share with others. Today, I am going to give you something special in return'. I happened to have my violin in my car ready for a performance at a charity concert that

---

4   This case was originally presented in the 'General Practitioner', *Adis International 1*, 13, August–September 1993, 17–18.

evening. I brought it into the therapy room and played Sonja a medley of
Hebrew and Gypsy melodies. Sonja flipped! 'Wow, Dr John', she said, 'that
was wonderful! I feel as though you have serenaded me'. 'And of course I
have', I responded quietly, 'And wouldn't it have been lovely if your Dad had
behaved as appropriately towards you when you were a child when he felt
his attraction towards you?'

Therapy has concluded after a further year – during which, Sonja
continued to change her dress much more freely, according to her fancy
rather than her need to maintain distance. She has also entered a relationship
with Les, 35 years, a computer analyst, who appears to listen to her and
respect her needs. Knives are no longer a cutting issue!

Discussion

Quite clearly, the structure in Sonja's family afforded her no protection: the
parents offered no nurturing and there was no education for adult life.
Possibly, if the abuse had been detected during Sonja's childhood, the
solution might have been a legal one – imprisonment of the perpetrator –
and not a therapeutic one. To arrange *meeting* with Sonja, I ensured that
boundaries were firm, that is therapeutic sessions were kept to a regular time,
place and frequency, and the mode of therapy was strictly conversational
with no physical touching, such as hugs, hands on the shoulder, etc.

I often 'listen' to what my body is telling me during therapy, such as
where I am tense, when I twitch, whether I am heavy or floating. This gives
me an intuition as to what may be occurring during conversation with clients.
During Sonja's early months of therapy, I sensed a multitude of powerful
feelings and so was able to *imagine the real* of her situation:

- Fear, experienced as a churning within my abdomen. As therapist, I
  shared with Sonja that her description of her murderous impulses
  were quite frightening to me and that it would take some time to
  build up a relationship of trust between us. I was comforted by the
  fact that her track record was good; she had not killed anyone as yet!
  I remarked also that I felt reasonably tough and able to withstand
  any verbal assault, any 'poison' that she might spew my way.

- Suffocation, experienced as a tightness in my throat. I told Sonja that
  I hoped the therapy room would become a safe place, an oasis,
  where she could 'speak the unspeakable'. I invited Sonja to 'tell her
  story' so that I could understand better 'what she was going through'.

- Rage, felt as an increasing tension within my limbs, accompanied by
  excitement and energy which I recognized as erotic attraction. Sonja

described how, when making love, she often considered stabbing her lovers full of holes. I commented that sometimes, when people are sexually abused as children, the 'wiring gets confused and sex and anger get all mixed up'. I encouraged Sonja to express her feelings through a medium which she enjoyed: writing. Sonja produced some essays quite worthy of the gothic horror fantasies of Edgar Allen Poe and Mary Shelley. Quite often, on reading her literature to me, Sonja would burst into gales of laughter and state that she would never do 'any of this stuff'.

○ Warmth, felt in an area near my heart, as a smile and in wrinkles surrounding my eyes. My statement acknowledging Sonja's softness and burning the photo which countered the 'family sham' appeared to enable Sonja to overcome her fear of sharing her sensitivity with me. The 'music lesson' perhaps provided a learning for Sonja that developing intimacy between therapist and client can be channelled appropriately and creatively.

On recounting this story one evening over a quiet drink, my friend Julian asked: 'Isn't it dangerous to do therapy when an attraction exists between you and your client?' My answer was then, and is now, definitely 'Yes!'…if therapy is conducted in isolation. The feelings of adult female survivors of sexual abuse often involve feelings of aggression and eroticism (Gunzburg 1991). The experience of male therapists frequently contains hidden patriarchal agendas which regard 'men's rights as being superior to those of women' (Leupnitz 1988). I converse regularly with professional peers whose prime interest is in contesting abuse by male perpetrators and countering patriarchal scripts. It is essential for we therapists to engage in peer, or formal, supervision so that we can ensure that we keep our clients (and ourselves) safe.

In inviting Sonja to *confirm* herself as a successful survivor of abuse, some useful questions to consider are: What were the patriarchal scripts influencing the attitudes and behaviours of Sonja's family? Were William's abusive actions overlooked because he was the 'Master' of the household and therefore above reproach? Was his violation regarded as the 'rather harmless foible' of an otherwise hard-working breadwinner? Did William regard Sonja as his property to be used for his gratification as he wished? Were women in this family to be sacrificed for the welfare of their men? What about nurturing? Did William consider this as Elspeth's 'job'? Were Elspeth's opinions regarding William's conduct towards Sonja discounted, not being worthy because they were a 'woman's point of view'? Were the secrecy and sham tools whereby 'men's rights' were protected in this family? The following essay is one of Sonja's descriptions of revenge on her father, William, who sexually abused her in her childhood.

Creeping up the stairs, lightly on my tiptoes, in the dead of night, I had the carving knife in my hand, ready to murder Dad. I was excited and yet trembling. I also felt like I was choking. There were curtains on the windows letting in the light. All was quiet. All I could hear were the night sounds. Everything was still peaceful. I carefully opened their bedroom door and crept in. I stood over them while they were sleeping. I remember when I was a girl, I had a dream where someone was standing over me, but I couldn't see their face. Someone was threatening me and now I was doing it back to them. I wanted to kill them and I felt creepy and wildly excited. I could knife both of them and finally get my revenge.

I was clutching the carving knife – the type chefs used, with a black handle and a very nasty blade – in my right hand. Dad woke up as he sensed some-one was there and I surprised him. He saw me and put his hand up to his forehead and tried to scramble away up the pillow, backing into the wall. I wasn't going to let him get away this time. I'd let him escape before, when he caused my breakdown by walking out on me and slinging me into chaos, into that black hole where my whole world had been pulled from under my feet and any sense of control and security I had had been carelessly thrown out the window as something unimportant. He was scared of me, as I now had the power, and I was going to taunt him with it and make him pay for all the confusion he had caused me. I could see that he was scared and I saw fear on his face. He was going to experience fear and the unknown, and the sexual control he had over me that was enough to send me into a feeling of rage-chaos, as I had experienced when I was little. I raised my hand and plunged my knife into his heart, repeatedly stabbing him, saying 'There, that's for you!' and 'You bastard!'. I was smiling to myself and felt madly out of control.

Working myself up into a mad frenzy (like an orgasm), I ripped his chest open like a savage dog after it has killed its prey and ripped his heart away from his body with my bare hands. I threw it to the ground like a possessed witch and laughed madly. I grabbed his two arms and ripped them out of their sockets. Being caught up in the excitement of the kill, I continued to hack his body up.

Mum was hysterical, her hands were up to her face, screaming. I spun around, screaming at her to shut up and threw my knife at her, straight into the middle of her throat. Her knees gave way and she fell to the floor. I chopped her up like a butcher when he is at the chopping block. I got a garbage bag from the kitchen and put their dismembered bodies into the bag and carried it downstairs like Santa carries his sack of toys over his shoulder. I threw them into the boot of the car and drove to Portsea back beach. I walked a little way into the bush and dug a shallow grave and dumped their remains there.

As I killed Dad, I experienced the ultimate orgasm, which I had been saving for him. I will never have another one so good. All my emotions of love and hate had flowed down that knife handle onto the blade and into Dad.

He did not have a heart.

I felt drained. There was nothing left

I felt??…what is it when a religious person purifies you???

There were many other literary rituals in which Sonja participated to contest her father's abuse. I asked her to write a copy of the Covenant which she believed best represented the contract that her father had forced upon her when she was a child. The Covenant is presented below:

An Act of Victoria

Agreement
1961
between the parties of – Kevin Reginald Pitman (adult)
                        – Sonja Esmeralda Pitman (minor)
drawn up by Kevin Reginald Pitman,

terms and conditions.

I, Sonja Esmeralda Pitman, hereby do agree upon the following terms and conditions:

- that I will not grow up and leave home
- that I will honour this agreement until death do we part, that is, upon my death.
- that I will not tell anyone of it's existence, and all denial of its existence will be made by Mr. Pitman
- that I, Sonja, will stand by my father, agreeing with whatever is said
- that I will be against Mum

- that I will only love one man, my Dad
- that I will not leave him emotionally for any other man
- that I will not have sex with any other man
- that I am bound to him
- that I will not form a sexual relationship or otherwise with any man
- that I will not leave him with Mum
- that I will not tell my Doctors
- that I am sworn to secrecy and upon telling, or if this covenant is broken, death will occur
- that I will squash any sexual arousal I may have towards the opposite sex
- that I vow to do as my father wishes, without question

Signed: Kevin Reginald Pitman

Signed: Sonja Esmeralda Pitman

Towards the end of Sonja's therapy, she told me that she had rewritten the Covenant as an adult. Sonja burnt the original Covenant and scattered the ashes to sea. A copy of the new Covenant is given below:

An Act of Parliament

of Victoria
1993

That I here revoke the previous act of 1961 between the parties of adult (Kevin Reginald Pitman) and minor (Sonja Esmeralda Pitman) as being void and unlawful. That all the terms and conditions are revoked as being unreasonable and unable to be carried out. That new terms and conditions be set and are as follows:

1) that I am free from the responsibilities of the previous past
2) that I am allowed to feel sexually aroused with a man of my choice to come to climax
3) that I can have erotic and interesting orgasms without feeling bad

4) that I love and respect my father's memory as a daughter (not as I would a former marriage partner) and that I will not hurt anyone

5) that I am no longer bound to keep my father's wishes/ pact alive (as he is dead)

6) that I no longer feel that it is impossible to break the covenant

7) that the covenant no longer exists

8) that I won't let your memory be a buffer between you and Mum

Signed: Kevin R. Pitman

Signed: Sonja E. Pitman

This document is now framed and hung on Sonja's wall!

At our final session, Sonja gave me a planter filled with linaria, candytuft and snapdragons, accompanied by the following letter:

Dear Dr. Gunzburg,

I'd like to say thank-you for all the help and love you have given me. I hope you have lots of good patients and lots of good jokes in the future.

Thank you

Goodbye

Love Sonja xox.

The developmental map

Two rabbis were entering the synagogue on the Day of Atonement. The first rabbi cried out: 'Oh, woe is me! Here I am, a wastrel in my youth, a fool during mid-life and a sinner in old age, and still I have not repented'. His companion replied: 'What are you doing raking muck? Rake it this way, rake it that way, it is always muck. Why rake muck when you could be stringing pearls for Heaven?'. (Buber 1947, p.130)

Families can be regarded as moving through normative developmental stages – courtship, marriage (whether formal or otherwise), birth of first and subsequent children, commencement of schooling, adolescence, children leaving home, retirement of spouse/s, death – and people can experience difficulties at any of these transitional points (Minuchin 1974). Moreover, there are many potential crises during the development of a family...illness, death, divorce, redundancy, war, migration – which can add to a person's struggle. Clients who request therapy often consider, as do their therapists, that their conflicts are deeply embedded within the muck of the past, arising from a stagnation at one of these developmental stages. They therefore often expect an intensive archaeological dig through the layers of Time to uncover what has kept them stuck at which developmental stage. The common understanding is that if only the problem can be discovered, the solution will inevitably follow.

I believe a more positive metaphor for encouraging psychological healing for adult survivors of abuse is to regard therapy as a quest for pearls to string for Heaven. Whilst an understanding of the contexts in which problems arose can be useful in framing solutions, the therapist's ability to increase the survivors' agency within their own lives and join them in the hunt for forgotten treasures and hidden resources is essential. This task is not such an easy one. Clients who seek help often expect their therapists to come up with a quick fix and a certain cure. This may be partly a reflection of cultural influences: that in our Western technological society, *doing* is much more highly valued over *being*. Getting to the goal is much more encouraged than participating in the journey. We therapists, however, can invite our clients into a conversational journey during which they can gradually tell their story and be heard respectfully. By searching for resources used at various developmental stages, clients can be encouraged to use those same resources to overcome their current difficulties.

Case 2H: Yeah, toffees![5]

October, 1992: Dennis 56 years, Patricia, 47, Nuela, 18, Donagh, 15 and Michael, 11, were standing nervously in my waiting-room, awaiting our first meeting. It was five days before Christmas and I offered them all a toffee of their choosing. Michael, sporting a cheeky grin, was the only one who accepted. The family told me quite a lengthy story of struggle. Dennis, unemployed, and Patricia, an invalid pensioner, had divorced six years previously, with Patricia remaining the custodial parent. Patricia described her ex-husband as a workaholic and this had led to the gradual emotional death of their marriage. Dennis agreed that he had put too much effort into his career and that, with the wisdom of hindsight, he would do things

---

5   This case was originally presented in the 'General Practitioner', *Adis International 1*, 7, June 1993, 10–11.

differently. Formerly employed in the fuel industry, he had endured two
significant business losses during the recession years of 1991–2 which had
created great financial strain. He was now training for a vocation in the real
estate field. Patricia said that three years earlier she had witnessed an episode
of shooting at a car during which a man was murdered. Since that time,
Patricia had received a series of threatening letters and harassing telephone
calls. She thought that they had been from the perpetrators, who were trying
to intimidate her (successfully!) from giving evidence against them. Six
months ago, Patricia had experienced a nervous breakdown, been diagnosed
a paranoid schizophrenic, certified and admitted to a mental institution for
two weeks. She settled on anti-psychotic medication and the malevolent
communications had ceased. I commented that perhaps Patricia had now
regained her safety. Her tormentors must have believed that, with a diagnosis
of 'craziness' against her, she would pose no threat in the witness stand.
Patricia agreed.

Two months before her hospitalization, Patricia had shifted into her own
accommodation because she felt that she needed space to calm down. The
children went to live with their father. Patricia said that she was now well,
was not taking any medication and wanted to reconstitute the family as it
was previously. Nuela and Donagh said that they preferred to live with their
father. Michael wanted to reside with them both. This was the family's
current dilemma.

Both Nuela and Donagh appeared down-hearted and said that this was
because, at Christmas time, theirs was not a 'normal' family living under one
roof. I replied that I did not know what a normal family was. Although theirs
was not a 'traditional' family, it was a pretty 'ordinary' family; almost one in
two families in Australia now living in a situation where the parents were
divorced/separated. I asked Nuela and Donagh if they wanted to have
traditional families themselves. They replied 'yes'. I asked Donagh if he
would go out with Dennis for a meal and discuss the mistakes he had made,
and would Nuela discuss with Patricia a 'woman's view' of why the
separation had occurred. Perhaps the parents would obtain consolation in
teaching the experience learnt from their errors and so help Nuela and
Donagh to avoid the same pitfalls.

I turned to Michael, saying that I had not forgotten him but that we had
been more occupied in discussing 'adult stuff' with his parents and elder
sister and brother. Now it was his turn. 'You look very much like a guy who
knows a good deal when he encounters one. You were the only person to
accept a toffee! You must know how to treat yourself. There has been so
much sadness and so little fun for all of you for so long. Would you be the

agent for fun for this family and plan a family activity that you would be sure that you would all enjoy?' (Michael and I left the room for a moment to secretly toss around some suggestions. We agreed that the family would probably all relish an outing to the new Science-Works Museum at Spotswood).

Discussion

This family's struggles seem to have commenced around the time of the divorce some years earlier. Remembering some ideas from the Structural Map, mentioned previously, both Dennis and Patricia acknowledged that Dennis's devotion to his vocation had weakened their marital bond and probably led to their divorce. I noted what my body was telling me, well into the first session: my forearm and neck muscles were tense and my fists and jaw were clenched. I usually carry my anger in this fashion and my hunch was that my posture signalled my reaction to a great deal of resentment within the family. (In fact, I was to learn later, during my own therapy, that the tension in my jaw muscles did not represent 'anger' but rather 'frustration'. In my family of origin, expression of anger was taboo and whenever anyone wanted to be angry it was usually expressed through clenched teeth. This enabled me to *imagine the real* of this family, that I was detecting the frustration with which various family members were struggling: Nuela and Donagh both were mourning the loss of their 'traditional family' at Christmas and seemed not yet to have spoken of their grief). There certainly had been many stressors, beside the marital split: the financial losses, Dennis's unemployment, Patricia's violation and her subsequent mental distress. Therapy, which continued fortnightly over three months, focused on expressing some of this anger and disappointment at shattered dreams, presenting the divorce as an ordinary event in today's society with which many families coped well and found a different sort of reward and increasing the parental support for Nuela and Donagh who appeared to be affected most. I also felt a fullness within my chest, which I recognised as admiration for this family. I was able to *confirm* Dennis's dedication to the children and his developing awareness, albeit in hindsight, of his errors and Patricia's obvious concern that family life proceed more easily. I endeavoured, where possible, to praise this family for their efforts. Finally, I detected a twinkle in my eyes and a warm smile for Michael – who knew a good toffee when it was offered to him. I highlighted his sense of fun as a resource, about which the family had forgotten in their hard times, to add lightness to the family. Six months later, Dennis is employed and all children visit Patricia regularly.

Case 21: The clerk

June, 1992: Harry, 52 years, a government clerk, who presented himself as a friendly man, willing to do anything for anybody else, told me of the bitterness and resentment that he had experienced over the past few months and requested a doctor's certificate for three months leave of absence from his employment so that he could 'get his act together'. In fact, I had seen Harry about four years previously to help him resolve some conflicts with colleagues at work (Gunzburg 1991, pp.116–117).

Harry told a heavy story. His father had had an affair whilst his mother was pregnant with Harry and, three months after the birth, she commenced lifelong residence in a mental institution. Harry was certain that his father's extramarital activities had contributed to this event. Harry had been raised from infancy by his mother's sister. He had been separated from his biological brother and sister with whom he now had little contact. He had been married and divorced twice. During his first marriage, Harry had lived with his in-laws and, apparently, his wife had had an affair with another family member with her family's covert consent. Harry's second spouse was an epileptic who appeared to have adopted a 'sick' role to Harry's 'carer' role before their split. Harry was endeavouring to remain in contact and to father the two children of this union as well as possible.

Harry said that he enjoyed writing short stories and pencil drawing. I invited him to script an account, perhaps accompanied by a picture, detailing some of the events that may have led to his emotional struggles, and gave him a week's rest from work. Harry shared his compositions at our next weekly meeting:

> I didn't know my biological mother until I was twenty-one years of age. I was brought up by my uncle and aunt (my mother's sister and her husband).
>
> I can only assume, by my mother's kind nature, that she would have been a very loving and caring person. Unfortunately, I cannot say the same for my natural father. In my dealings, or association that I had with him, he was a very hard and heartless sort of person. He had my mother committed to a mental asylum in Adelaide just after I was born, so as I am had to believe, to marry another woman with whom he had been having a relationship for some time prior to my birth.
>
> I would have had a family relationship with my sister and brother, which I did not have with my uncle and aunt. So I suppose I missed out on the family love as a unit. Presently my relationship with my brother is fairly close. My sister, she is much more distant, there is no communication with her as she has gone her own way.

I have tried to analyse the situation and I really cannot say that I would have been any different or better than I am now. I can only say that I feel that I was cheated on by our separation, as I never grew up with my brother or sister.

I cannot complain about my up-bringing as I feel sure my father, in particular, would not have given me the morals or principles that I have in my life.

I know he would not have encouraged me to remain with my religion as he said to me, and so did his 'wife' on a few occasions when I stayed with them on school holidays, and I quote: 'If you come and live with us, you won't be going to your silly Catholic church or school. You will go to a proper school'.

'What if?'... I really don't know, but I do feel as though I have missed out on something; a proper family life, mother, father, brother, sister. I hope this makes sense.

As we talked about Harry's essay, I noted that I was furrowing my brow, wrinkling my nose, pouting my lips and tensing my calf muscles. I recognised these signs as my dislike of Harry and, as he had communicated nothing too outrageous to me, I decided to discuss my reactions with one of my peers before the next session. Two points came to the fore:

1. That Harry had asked for three months rest from work. I seemed to be favouring the patriarchal notion that Harry should 'tough it out' and not take the 'weaker and lazier' option of stopping work. My colleague suggested that perhaps I was working too hard at that particular moment and needed to assess my own leisure needs more accurately.

2. That Harry appeared to be asking me to 'care' for him much more than perhaps I perceived his situation warranted. In my family of origin, I had assumed the role of 'carer' to much of my family at the cost of much teenage and young adult enjoyment (a past conversation which my uncle, my father's brother, had in Perth with his son affirmed this situation for me. My uncle had said to my cousin rather brusquely: 'John did not need to leave Western Australia and travel to live in Melbourne. He could have taken over Dr. Stork's old practice'. Dr. Stork had been general practitioner to our entire family!) I had also, around the time, adopted a friendly style of relating to hide my loneliness within. My colleague invited me to consider whether Harry's request was triggering off some of my own resentment towards, and rejection of, his therapeutic

requirements. As important, was Harry having this same effect within his social and vocational network: creating a distance between himself and his associates and increasing his feelings of acrimony?

At our next meeting, Harry and I introduced the theme of 'carer/cared for' roles within families. Had Harry missed out on the caring and emotional nourishment that he required in childhood, due to his father's rejection and mother's hospitalization, and adopted the 'carer' role, hoping that by loving others they would love him in return? Had others detected the mournful solitude underlying Harry's cheery façade and made moves to distance themselves from him? We discussed ways of 'caring for self' – nourishing food, warm baths, massage, relaxation, walks in the park, comfortable sleep, music, movies, writing, drawing. I admired Harry for his strength in enduring the abuses of his father and first wife's family and his ability to accept the misfortunes that had befallen him and look towards his future. We talked about the possible images of abuse revealed within his picture – the spider's web, the grave stone, the fallen cross, the bird's talons, the tree bare of fruit and leaves, the storm with thunder and lightning. We also discussed the symbols of hope that were represented in Harry's picture – love, spirituality, light, the search to discover what 'Life is', the olive branch of peace, an invitation to enter the closed door and move on in his life, and how to find the key to unlock that door and progress through it. Harry required only three weeks away from work. He said that he was regaining his confidence and an internal sense of calm. I asked him what had made the difference. Harry said that when he had composed his description and picture of his life, they had affirmed for him that he *had* come through hard times successfully and that perhaps there were better times to be had ahead. Therapy lasted five weeks in all and I made sure that my next few weekends were restful ones!

Discussion

Harry appeared to have missed out on a good deal of nurturing in his early years due to his mother's mental institutionalization, and to have experienced a great deal of deception at the hands of his family. This case illustrated vividly for me that when we therapists are trying to *imagine the real* circumstances of our clients, we must be aware of how their situation mirrors or impinges on ours. I felt that Harry was asking me to carry him emotionally over a long distance. This is an appropriate request for a client to make of a therapist, but I experienced Harry adopting the same dependent role in a manner similar to other family members in my youth. Had I not sought peer supervision, I would have had little hope of *meeting* with Harry. I was also reminded that I utilized the same tactics of 'being pleasant' to others to hide my own sense of seclusion. Having sorted out what was 'my stuff' and what was 'his stuff', I was more able to highlight his resource of writing and drawing, inviting Harry to reflect on what he had missed during his youth. A discussion of 'carer/cared for' roles proved beneficial to us both, and some further questions that might have proved useful to *confirm* Harry as a person growing towards independence are: Was Harry's yearning to love others fuelled by patriarchal mythology, that men and women are incomplete without one another, that people who need people are the luckiest people in the world? (a co-operative approach might be expressed as people who are able to care for themselves are more likely to choose partners with whom they can enjoy life mutually). Is the 'sick' role one of the recognized ways that women can gain attention from their men in a patriarchal community? Was the incestuous affair between Harry's first wife and her relative grounded within a patriarchal script, that women are property to be shared between men within the family? (the possibility of my being influenced by the patriarchal attitudes of 'over-valuing men's work' and 'under-valuing men's emotional needs' has been noted).

The psychodynamic map

The greater part of our minds can be considered as being involved in unconscious processes. Undesirable events happen to us during our development, often early in childhood, which can be regarded as being repressed into our unconscious. These repressed events can affect our subsequent thinking and behaviour as adults. Part of our life-process as adults can be considered as gaining insight, recovering details of the repressed events so that their influence on us can be modified, and making freer choices in our lives.

Case 2J: Going under[6]

June, 1992: Lesley, 50 years, manager of a sportswear store, and Greta, 26, a clerical worker in an advertising firm, sat in my room quietly. As I drew their family's genogram, I noted that Lesley was trembling and Greta appeared sombre. Lesley told me of her terror over the past five days that had prevented her from doing almost every activity. She had asked Greta to accompany her as she felt she could not travel on her own.

---

6   This case was originally presented in the 'General Practitioner', *Adis International 1, 2,* March 1993, 10–11.

Lesley continued to speak for them both. She related how, in 1980, she had undergone radical mastectomy for breast cancer. In 1983, she and her husband, Geoffrey, now 55, an advertising consultant, had divorced. Lesley described Geoffrey as an 'uncommunicative' man who seemed to be preoccupied with his own life, without much time to spend with the rest of the family. Nonetheless, after the separation, Geoffery had contributed regularly to the financial welfare of his children and Lesley had been pleased with the way that Greta and Ted, now 23 and a motorbike mechanic, had both continued an amicable relationship with their father. Ted appeared to be a bit like Geoffery now: he did not seem to be too bothered by his mother's distress and had offered her a vote of confidence, describing Lesley as a 'tough lady' who had been able to surpass many obstacles in the past. Lesley told me how an aunt had been hospitalized for depression many times during her mid-life and Lesley wondered if she was also 'going mad'. My thoughts were that Lesley had experienced a 'roller coaster' existence over the past decade or so and that she may be reacting to remembered emotions of these events, long suppressed within the unconscious part of her psyche and now stirring to be addressed. Having become rather cautious in nature during my career as therapist, I also wondered if there had been episodes of abuse in Lesley's past that might be affecting her now. Because of the severity of Lesley's panic, and Greta's presence, I did not broach the subject of possible past violations during this first session; I did not want to encroach on Lesley's sense of privacy and concentrated on setting up a safe, comfortable therapeutic environment in which we could proceed.

I was admiring that the family had done well since the illness and divorce and queried which event had created the most stress. 'Oh, it was the mastectomy', replied Lesley, 'that was an awful time for all of us. I was so sick after the chemotherapy and the kids were so worried. But it was the thing that convinced me that my marriage with Geoffery was finished. Though he was obviously concerned that I should recover, he made no moves to help me in any practical or emotionally supportive way. I don't think he stopped concentrating on his business for a moment'. We continued to talk about the mastectomy and Lesley's relative sense of isolation within the family at that time. How had the children, then both adolescents, coped with their anxieties? Had they known what was happening? Had Lesley, Greta, and Ted shared their fears when the teenagers were faced with their mother's death and Lesley was confronted by Eternity? Had they comforted each other? Would Lesley and Greta both treat themselves to a restaurant and discuss how they felt about their fears now? Did they need to comfort each other during Lesley's current stress?

'Fear sometimes eventuates from crises way back', I remarked. 'When my daughter suffered meningitis six years ago, my own fears resulting from my own brush with death from meningitis at eighteen months of age surfaced (Gunzburg 1991). I had to work those feelings through to a resolution during the therapy I was undertaking at that time (I had telephoned my mother to let her know about my daughter's progress and she had said to me: 'You know, you almost died of meningitis when you were a toddler. You were hospitalized for ten days'. I had completely forgotten this event, although the Disney characters painted on the infants' ward of the hospital had seemed strangely familiar when I had been a medical student there. My therapist had said to me: 'If you almost died of meningitis at eighteen months of age, at that age you would have detected the feelings of your parents, the doctors and nurses, their fears and anxieties for your well-being. Having experienced these feelings when you were pre-verbal, you would have had difficulty labelling them and discussing them as an adult'. I had burst into tears during the therapy session and wept for half an hour. An ancient, primitive insecurity – my constant companion for over forty years – had been named and I was able to let it go). I can understand, Lesley, your being concerned at being cursed like your aunt but enough has happened to you in your life to scare you out of your wits. We have only just met but I cannot detect the slightest bit of madness in you'. Lesley unleashed a whoosh of breath as though an enormous force had gushed from her.

The next week, Lesley told me that she and Greta had dined and conversed about their past fears. Greta felt no further need to attend. Lesley asserted that she would come alone. Her terror gone, she had assumed ordinary routines. I was impressed by Lesley's resilience. I asked her: 'What has made the difference?' Lesley replied that there were two significant points: First, my account of meningitis seemed to have created impact. Lesley had not realized that such episodes could cause sustained unconscious influence. She recalled almost drowning at the beach when she was two. Second, Lesley had contemplated other 'mad' relatives in the family, particularly one of her mother's 'wild drunkard' brothers, now deceased, who had sexually abused her when she was five, and had fully realized her overwhelming fear of going crazy. My statement that she did not appear to be going mad had created impact. I encouraged Lesley to see *Back to the Future*, a film which reflects therapeutic method: going back in time, re-working 'unfinished' situations and using new skills learnt within the current moment. I also invited her to write a letter to her abuser, expressing her adult feelings. Some further sessions were spent discussing the concept of 'patriarchal male entitlements': had Lesley's uncle, when intoxicated, perceived her as a child who was to be the object for his pleasure rather than a person to protect? Did Geoffery assess his work needs to be greater than those of Lesley when she was afflicted with breast cancer? Perhaps, when Lesley and Geoffery had first met, Geoffery had appeared to be the 'strong, quiet, dependable' stereotype of a husband and Lesley had hoped that he would offer her a much different experience to that which she had encountered with her irresponsible and undisciplined uncle. What observations would Lesley have to make about her future potential partners to ascertain as early as possible whether they were abusive or not?

Discussion

I listened quietly to Lesley as she told her story of struggle. It was this act of quiet attention that enabled client and therapist to *meet*. From Lesley's trembling, her clearly expressed fears of developing 'mid-life' madness and Greta's sombre attitude, I was able to *imagine the real* situation of both. Here were mother and daughter co-operating as allies and battling against the odds. The main effector of change appears to have been my exploring the unconscious issues that influenced Lesley, and shared experiences from the therapist's own life emphasised the powerful influence of unconscious mechanisms. The therapist then explored ways family members supported each other in the past, that is, at the time of the mastectomy, did mother and teenagers comfort each other's fears? Lesley and Greta shared their fears and affirmed their bond. Lesley stated that her fears had fled and declared that my highlighting of unconscious processes, assurance that her mind was sound and recalling her uncle's abuse were effectors of change. Cinema was used to illustrate flow of therapy. Letter writing was utilized to contest the uncle's abuse and *confirm* Lesley's personhood as a successful survivor of abuse. The focus shifted towards Lesley's relationships and patriarchal patterns underlying her past violation and Geoffery's neglect, further *confirming* Lesley's ability to act as an advocate for her own future. Questions were explored, such as: Did Lesley choose Geoffrey, a withdrawn man, as the opposite of the alcohol-abusing uncle who sexually violated her in childhood? How might Lesley choose a more emotionally disciplined yet communicative partner if she so wished?

Note the therapeutic process I have tried to illustrate here:

○ During our *meeting*, Lesley offered her description and construction of the problem: that her feelings were a measure of her developing insanity.

- I *imagined the real* of Lesley's situation and invited her to consider that her feelings were more to do with unconscious memories of crises and abuses than any constitutional deficit.

- A conversation now took place *between* us. Lesley's view was deconstructed, connecting her current emotions with the disruptions initially experienced during family struggles, and she was encouraged to think about unconscious processes.

- Lesley introduced new information: she remembered her near-death through drowning and an uncle's sexual abuse. Lesley became calmer and commenced to plan new directions for the future.

- Lesley's changes were affirmed and mother and daughter were *confirmed* as persons able to nourish one another and utilize each other as a resource.

- Further *confirmation* of personhood continued. Lesley viewed a film which described how therapy could help resolve 'unfinished' situations. She was invited to write a letter to her abuser contesting his violations. During conversation between Lesley and me, the information gained from these tasks could be used in the mutual reconstruction of a new communal context within which Lesley could examine her feelings towards personal relationships. Through overcoming her mistrust of her male intimates abusing and/or depriving her, and realising that there are ways to contest the attitudes of patriarchal men, Lesley hopefully will learn to deepen her current friendships.

The communicational map

Symptoms, thoughts and behaviours can be regarded as pieces of information – as metaphors – about what is happening within the family (Haley 1984).

When people say that they have a communication problem, often they are saying that they do not know how to interpret accurately what their intimate partner is telling them. Their partner may state: 'It is cold!' then, thirty minutes later, flare up in a temper: 'You never do anything I ask of you! I wanted you to throw another log on the fire!' Or they may say: 'I am happy', leaving their listener to wonder whether it is their job, the state of their relationship, the evening meal or the leisure activity in which they are presently occupied that is rewarding to them at that moment.

In these circumstances, therapy becomes a conversation to facilitate the analytic skills of clients in clarifying communication and receiving feedback about what has been said. What exactly happened in the situation being considered? What was said, and who said it? What was the response to such a statement? What happened next? Therapists, by asking these questions and by tracking the process of events during interactions within a family, peer or social group, can model for clients how to do the same.

When people say that they have a communication problem, often they are saying that they do not know how to place what their intimate partner is telling them within a certain context. A spouse may say: 'My stomach is full of concrete!' If he or she has previously been diagnosed as schizophrenic, this statement may be taken as evidence of delusion, but it might also be a comment on the spouse's home cooking just consumed! Parents may claim: 'Our adolescent is a disgrace, missing several days of school each month and showing us up as bad parents'. The school refusal, however, may be due to a grief reaction to the recent death of a grandparent, an imminent marital split or the arrival of a cousin who has come to stay long-term – with resultant loss of privacy. The comment or behaviour, then, can be regarded as a symbol of what is happening within the clients' internal experience or within their wider interactional sphere.

Therapists can explore the various contexts with clients to clarify exactly which one applies to the troublesome behaviour. A statement made to the spouse of the schizophrenic can open a way for new information: 'I can see that you are concerned as to the mental deterioration of your partner, has anything else happened to alert you?' A genogram compiled with the family's help can offer explanations other than teenage rebellion for the school refusal. Often, giving clients the idea that dialogue and behaviours can occur in more than one context, and that the meaning of such words or actions can vary with each context, can be enough in itself to induce change.

When people say that they have a communication problem, often what they are saying is that what their intimate is telling them does not seem to fit with the way their partner appears to be feeling at the time: 'Of course I want to go to the party with you! (grunt, growl, snarl)' is a mixed message that conveys both compliance and defiance. The receiver of the message frequently ends up feeling confused, unable to respond and emotionally labile.

The task of therapists here can be considered to ensure that communication between clients and their intimates is congruent; that the words spoken match the underlying feelings. Open-ended questions are most useful in making overt exactly what it is that participants wish to express, for example How did you feel when you said (or heard) that? What are you experiencing right at this moment? What do you notice about your partner when she/he says that? Comments by therapists about body language can open the way for change: 'You say that you want to go to the party but I note that your right hand is clenched and your voice sounds tense. Is there anything else that you would rather do?'

I tell the following stories to illustrate the intricacies of human communication described above, particularly when clients are embroiled in conflict over what a word or sentence means.

Case 2K: The lie[7]

During April 1988, Thelma, 43 years, told me of her guilty secret in her strong, Cockney accent: 'When m'husband left me, I felt so bad. I told everyone that I was dyin' of cancer. That was wrong, wasn't it, to tell such a lie like that? I am religious. I shouldn't of told a lie like that' 'How did you feel when your husband left you?' I asked Thelma. 'Like I was dyin'', she replied, 'it hurt me so bad I felt like I was dyin''. 'So you really did not tell such a lie, did you?' I responded, 'Perhaps what you really did was to express to others just how bad it felt for you, without enduring their taunts that you had a broken marriage'.

Thelma's sense of guilt was less after two further sessions and we were able to move on to expressing her grief and anger at the way the marriage had ended (How do you feel about it? What aspect is unfinished for you? Which aspect do you wish to tackle in this session?)

Discussion

This is a nice example of how individuals can confuse literal communication with metaphoric, or descriptive, communication (Gunzburg and Stewart 1994). Thelma appeared to be punishing herself with guilt for her perceived transgression of the internalized injunction 'Thou shalt not lie!' I invited her to consider the context of her story that she was dying of cancer. Rather than a literal untruth, it could be regarded more as a metaphor of how she felt when her husband left her. It had conveyed the depth of her pain whilst sparing her the feeling of shame in having to tell others about her 'failed' relationship. This brief interaction involved all aspects of Buber's *genuine dialogue* that we have been considering. Thelma and I were able to *meet* in a safe and comfortable environment and, gaining information as to what happened to give rise to her guilt, I was able to *imagine the real* of her situation. I invited Thelma to perceive her lie as a vivid description of her emotions at her husband's departure, rather than a literal untruth. This can be considered an act of *inclusion*, encouraging Thelma to view herself less harshly. I value

---

7   This case was originally presented in *Patient Management 14*, 8, August 1990, 101–8.

an easier, less fundamentalist, way of viewing the world and, in sharing this with Thelma, endeavoured to include both of us within this framework. Finally, Thelma, in expressing her feelings of anger and sorrow rather than guilt and shame, can be regarded as *confirming* herself as a person able to experience healthier emotions rather than ones which imprison her.

Case 2L: That ol' black magic[8]

Another story about Lesley and Marnie (see Case 1F:A hidden message, p.20). Lesley was concerned that she was going to bash her daughter and do her an injury. 'She is always nagging me about AIDS!', Lesley complained of Marnie, 'She keeps asking me: "Have you washed this? Have you cleaned this? Do you get AIDS from touching this, Mummy?" Fifty bloody times a day! I am really going to belt her one!'

When Marnie attended the next session with Lesley, I asked her if she knew why I had wanted to see her. Marnie replied that her Mum could tell me what the problem was and that she would cover her ears with her hands so that she would not hear that word. Marnie did so and Lesley said: 'It is that worry about AIDS'. Marnie uncovered her ears and I told her that although Mum had revealed to me that word, it would be better if Marnie were to describe it herself to me; Did it have a specific colour? Marnie replied that it was black, and shaped her fingers into a ball. 'So it is a black ball', I commented, 'Large or small?' 'A little one', Marnie replied.

We kept on talking for a while about these sinister little black balls that could keep bouncing into our lives at will, getting into people's way and causing a lot of trouble. 'I wonder how you could protect yourself whenever a little black ball bounced your way?', I pondered. Marnie thought that if she went out and bought a red jumper it might help protect her. It was such a bright colour and she could wear it to bed to keep her safe at night. 'And red is the colour of blood, of life, I added. Marnie nodded. It turned out that Marnie had a penchant for vampire movies and I noted that she was wearing a small gold cross on a necklace. Crosses were great for keeping vampires away; perhaps they would work on little black balls also? Perhaps Marnie could polish her cross regularly and keep it nice and shiny? As we discussed this idea, I thought: 'Whoops! Am I offering a training course in obsessive-compulsive behaviour here?!'

Three months later, Lesley told me that Marnie had not mentioned AIDS since that session. She had chosen a red tracksuit as the new item of clothing to wear every now and then and occasionally Marnie would polish her cross to ensure that it retained its golden glow.

---

8   This case was originally presented in Gunzburg 1991, pp.211–212.

Discussion

Lesley can still be regarded as viewing her parenting of Marnie within an I–It position: Lesley considering herself as an 'It', a 'bad mother' who was raising Marnie, also an 'It', an 'irrationally fearful child'. Lesley also appeared to think that Marnie's concern about AIDS reflected her own hypochondriacal worries. (In fact, Lesley was being more than an adequate mother, requesting help before she lashed out at Marnie). I *imagined the real* of Marnie's situation, that AIDS did communicate Marnie's fear, but of a different nature: fear of loss. Lesley, Marnie and their family were due to shift house away from neighbourhood friends and schoolmates within the month. Inviting Marnie to consider how the 'little black balls' disturbed her peace can be regarded as an act of *inclusion*, helping make this fear concrete and empowering Marnie to protect herself in a manner that appealed to her sense of play.

Case 2M The snob[9]

'It is my wife, Wendy, doctor', complained Bartholomew, 36 years, who managed several hairdressing salons. 'Whenever we party, and I socialize among guests, trying to build up my clientele, Wendy hangs back and does not mingle. They all think that she is a snob. It is bad for business'.

During a few weekly sessions with Wendy, 30, on her own, she told of the sexual abuse that her father had perpetrated on her between the ages of 4 and 14 years, after which she had left home. She had had a disastrous former marriage before she had met Bartholomew. They had two children, Nathan, 8, and Claire, 6. Although Wendy felt far more comfortable with Bartholomew than with her previous spouse, she held back sexually, had not told him about the incest, and felt intensely resentful that he pushed her into social contacts. She was petrified of strange men within groups.

A further joint session with this couple was spent in discussing Wendy's past. Her husband was more able to comprehend Wendy's reticence and they agreed that he would not leave her unaccompanied for lengthy periods at social gatherings. Bartholomew said that he had been frustrated by his wife's lack of sexual initiation, but could more understand her feelings and was willing to let her develop at her own pace.

At the last contact, some eighteen months later, this couple had entered a joint business venture where Wendy managed the administrative side of the arrangement, meeting his clients within a secure structure.

---

9   This case was originally presented in Gunzburg 1991, p.212.

Discussion

To Bartholomew, Wendy's 'distance' from the social group appeared to communicate aloofness and snobbery. To Wendy, her 'distance' seemed to be a measure of her fear of men. Understanding what each other experienced as 'distance' can be regarded as enabling Bartholomew to lessen his demands on Wendy to change and empowering Wendy to feel more supported and to participate in Bartholomew's world. In Buber's terminology, Wendy and Bartholomew (and I) can be considered as *meeting* and, through exploring the different experiences that the word 'distance' communicated for each of them, they were able to *include* each other within their world-view. They were then able to negotiate lifestyles that *confirmed* their own needs and their relationship with each other.

There is another story that I like to tell that demonstrates that words communicate very different meanings to adult and child: My daughter Rahel, 7, suffering from a greenstick fracture just acquired in the playground, was waiting in the school infirmary to be taken home. 'My daddy is a doctor', she said proudly to Matron. 'That is lovely, dear', Matron replied, 'What sort of doctor is he?' 'A kind one', was the reply.

The transgenerational map

Deborah Leupnitz (1988) considers the concept of *transgenerational* repetition of problems is very significant to therapy:

> We tend to repeat the emotional life of our forebears for two main reasons. The first is that what we experience is simply what we know best and what we assume to be universal. A man with a depressed mother unconsciously learns to associate femininity with depression. Similarly, women who are abused by men in childhood often grow up thinking that they deserve abuse. Such people are not doomed to reproduce the past forever, but without help of some type, they have an excellent chance of doing so. The second reason that we repeat is the effort to master experiences of childhood. The man with the depressed mother may have been engaged as her comforter as a child, but of course could not cure her depression. He may, however, believe that he can cure his fiancée of hers. The woman with the abusive father may feel about her abusive boyfriend, 'If only I can get this dangerous man to love me!' thereby mastering the situation in childhood when she could not protect herself from father... Another way of depicting this tendency to repeat the past is Gregory Bateson's passage from the Book of *Ezekiel* 'The fathers have eaten bitter fruit, and the children's

teeth are set on edge (18:2)'. Bateson pointed out that it is not so bad for the parents; they know what they ate. But the children who invariably suffer the effects of the bitter food do *not* know, and they will continue to take in what is sickening, believing that there is nothing else. (pp. 191–2).

Case 2N: The right sort of guidance?[10]

June, 1990: I had been seeing Geoff, 39 years, a part-time worker in a canteen, every two to three weeks for a couple of years to help him contain his feelings of anger. Geoff currently was distressed that his girlfriend, Myra, 36, unemployed, seemed so erratic in her behaviour. Geoff and Myra had shared accommodation for two years but had been arguing with increased ferocity over the past few months. The main focus of conflict appeared to be Myra's heroin addiction, present since her adolescence. Myra would admit herself into a rehabilitation centre but, on discharge, would quickly revert to her habit. Geoff would become infuriated and 'tell her off'. A fight would ensue and Myra would leave. Her last departure was six weeks previously when Myra had set up house with Tim, 45, her drug dealer.

Both Geoff and Myra had experienced great anguish in their past. Geoff's mother had died during his birth and his father, a jockey, had been killed in a riding accident when Geoff was three. After living with his grandparents for two years, Geoff had been raised to young adulthood within orphanages and foster homes. He remembered many fights with, and harsh disciplines from, his caretakers. Geoff had been a drifter for much of his life, being involved constantly in street brawling and seeking friendships among criminal associates. When twenty years old, Geoff had been caught and charged with armed robbery. He had served a five-year gaol term. On his release, Geoff had decided to 'go straight'. He started working in a series of unskilled jobs and paired up with Kim, 34, a clerical worker. Kim had left Geoff, and their three children who were all under five years of age, to live with a lover three years previously. Geoff had fostered them out successfully and had maintained regular contact with all of them. Myra had been physically abused by her father, had run away from home in her teens and had been involved in a series of bashings and rapes before she met Geoff. Geoff had hit Myra twice ('But never with my closed fist, Doc!', he asserted) during the two years that they had known each other. At our next joint meeting, Myra admitted that Geoff was 'a pretty decent bloke' and the best thing that had happened to her, but she had been frightened of him since

---

10 This case was originally presented in the 'General Practitioner', *Adis International 1*, 18, November 1993, 14–15.

the last time he had slapped her several weeks ago. I checked if Myra knew the address of a Women's Refuge should she require one and if she felt safe enough to continue the friendship with Geoff. Myra responded 'Yes' to both questions. She said that she had obtained therapy at her drug rehabilitation centre and did not wish to attend further sessions with Geoff.

I had continually affirmed Geoff for his sense of responsibility to his children and partner and restraint of his angry feelings, which he said verged on the 'murderous' at times. I had no doubt of his genuine affection for Myra and concern for her welfare. I wove the themes of 'traditional men's roles' into our therapeutic conversation. Geoff seemed to have learnt early that 'men need to battle each other to gain what they want' and that 'women need both protection and discipline from their male partners'.

I had asked Geoff: 'Do you think, underneath it all, that Myra expects you to be like her violent Dad? He was the model of manhood with which Myra grew up. He seems always to have treated her like a 'bad girl'. Perhaps Myra thinks that she can only have a friendship with you as the bad girl who always requires to be disciplined? And perhaps you feel your job is to give Myra guidance as to how to get the best out of her life? Myra's father seems to have resorted primarily to beating Myra as a method of correction. Are you falling into the same pattern? You have shown great commitment in supporting Myra and your kids, and you obviously want them to do well. On those occasions when you hit Myra, do you become 'a monster', just like her father? When she walks away from it all, do you get furious that she spurns your good advice, just like all those other women who have rejected you before? We adults all need to nurture each other and be nurtured at times. Sometimes, nurturers are most effective when they nourish their loved ones from a distance. They do not direct but, rather, let others learn from their own mistakes.' Geoff was quiet and looked thoughtful at the end of our session.

Over the next three months, there were some changes: Tim had been charged with trafficking drugs and gaoled, Myra had wanted to return to Geoff, Geoff had told Myra that he preferred her to live elsewhere but that he would be happy to see her regularly for lunch and a chat. This they did. Geoff currently has care of his son Benny, seven, and daughter Sally, five, and says he is enjoying single parenthood. Myra has entered a drug rehabilitation centre once more, and Geoff says that when they do meet there is no arguing or fighting.

Discussion

The transgenerational repetition in Geoff's life appears to be centred around the theme of 'rejection': his mother died during his childbirth, he lost his grandmother as carer when he entered an orphanage and his wife left for another partner. Perhaps Geoff views women within an 'I–It' position, believing them to be 'quitters who are never there for their men'? Perhaps, with the 'right sort of guidance', he can educate Myra to stay and not leave him? Geoff becomes enraged whenever Myra does depart and he lashes out at her. Myra was battered mercilessly by her father. Perhaps she regards herself within an 'I–It' position, anticipating that all she is worthy of is continued abuse from her boyfriends? I comment that Geoff's response to Myra's perceived abandonment simulates the father's violation. We discuss some patriarchal scripts that may be influencing Geoff's perception of his masculinity. This can be considered an act of *inclusion*: I, as a man, acknowledging responsibility to contest male violence towards women. I suggest that 'parenting/nurturing' can follow a different course: one can love intimates from a distance in a manner that empowers and fosters independence. Geoff and Myra set up a different social arrangement – one in which they can *meet* – by negotiating a friendship whilst living in separate residences and Geoff takes over the personal care of his children.

Aftermath

I did not see Geoff for many months. He returned to therapy just after Tim's release from gaol, and he was fuming! Myra had stopped approaching Geoff and had gone to live with her former drug dealer. 'I am going to get that hoon!', Geoff swore. 'He is just using Myra, offering her drugs for favours. I am going to get a couple of my mates and break his kneecaps with a baseball bat!' I could not shift Geoff from his resolve. He disappeared for three months. As he had no telephone number, I sent off a letter expressing my concern as to his safety but received no reply. The general practitioner who had initially referred him contacted me and asked if I had seen Geoff recently. I said 'No'. The practitioner told me that the police had found Geoff dead in his flat that previous evening, his arms covered with needle marks. 'But Geoff did not use drugs', I commented, 'there was not the slightest indication that he was doing so'. 'That is what I think also', continued the practitioner, 'but the authorities have decided to treat this as just another accidental overdose. Geoff's children have gone to live with their mother. The case is closed!'.

Some further questions to invite male clients to consider the issues regarding male violence towards women, and *confirm* themselves as responsible men, might be: Was Myra's heroin addiction an attempt to gain a sense of internal comfort and fun that she had been denied in her childhood due to her father's abuse; or was it a means of 'anaesthetic' against the memories of the abuse; or was it an attempt to 'belong' to the drug culture? What patriarchal myths had Geoff been taught in his family of origin: that men are the bosses; that men are obliged to fight each other for their rights; that women are to be cared for; that women need direction from their male partners; that it is permitted to hit women as long as a man doesn't use a closed fist or a weapon; that women are possessions to be fought over?

The analytic – 'reductive-into-parts' map

Were I to write my largest book, it would be one incorporating mistakes I have made over my many years as a therapist. However, I am told by my publishers that such a book would not sell! Most readers want to be informed about successes rather than errors. It is probably true, however, that, whilst I am always rather tentative about what is effective in creating change during the therapeutic conversations I have with clients, experience has given me a fairly useful guide as to what doesn't work during the therapy in which I participate. Generally, my mistakes occur when I slip into a rigid role, relate to the client in stereotypical fashion and seduce myself with my own cleverness into thinking that 'I know what to do' rather than exploring the client's expertise to discover solutions.

Whenever I err, I am usually guilty of linear, analytical or reductive-into-parts thinking. Such thinking is not of itself inherently harmful. I would not want anyone to remove my inflamed appendix in any other manner, that is consider all the information available, make a diagnosis, find the offending organ and whip it out quick-smart! Psychological healing, however, utilizes a lateral, synthetic, holistic approach, that is being able to step outside of a problem situation and consider it from a number of angles. When I think linearly, I fall into the trap of thinking that every event has a single, definite and discoverable cause, and if only I can behave in a certain way, or search diligently and long enough, the 'Truth will out!' This may lead to discounting or trivializing the client and what Buber would call *mismeeting* between myself and my clients.

The three case histories below detail examples of mistakes made which upset the *meeting* that had been created previously and resulted in distance between my clients and I. Descriptions as to how my clients and I countered the effects of my mistakes are also offered.

Case 20: The actor

March, 1993: Peta, 28 years, trained as an actor, described the depression that had stalked her for the past three years, resulting in her obtaining an invalid pension. Peta had been raised within a family in which her father Dick had verbally abused everyone else and her mother Marlene appeared to have used Peta, the youngest child, as a target for her resentment at Dick's mistreatment. A male family friend had sexually abused Peta when she was fourteen and her brother James, a heroin addict and elder than Peta by two years, had hung himself five years previously. Peta was also experiencing difficulties in her relationship with Rowan, 31, a well-known Melbourne stand-up comedian, whom she described as discounting and emotionally depriving. Rowan had decided to give Peta 'the flick' when she had asked for a commitment to monogamy within their relationship. The early sessions of weekly therapy were spent in expressing the grief related to James' suicide, contesting the violation in adolescence and discussing patriarchal dynamics. Would Marlene have treated Peta so badly if Dick had contributed safety and nurturing to the family? Had James killed himself to escape Dick's abuse? Despite her anger, Marlene had always 'been there' for Dick and Peta appeared to have copied this pattern of 'caring for her male partners no matter what'. How could Peta change? After four months, Peta seemed to trust me more and said that she and Rowan were talking about reconciliation. I invited Peta to bring Rowan to a joint session. This she did the subsequent week. I thought that the meeting went well, my having engaged Rowan into therapy by sharing our ideas about our respective careers and the creativity involved. We had agreed to meet as a threesome the following week. At this meeting, however, Peta, who attended on her own, expressed her fury at me, claiming that I had focused the whole of the last session on Rowan and had ignored her completely. I felt overwhelmed by the intensity of Peta's anger and asked if she would allow me a week to consider how I might have contributed to her distress. Between sessions I sought peer review. My colleagues all suggested that I had discounted Peta, permitting myself to be seduced into 'paying homage to the famous Rowan' rather than treating him as a 'guest at Peta's therapy'. When Peta returned a week later, I thanked her for giving me the opportunity to collect and present my thoughts. I acknowledged that I had disregarded her needs during the joint session, yielding to the temptation to worship Rowan's and my own celebrity. I believed that in so doing, I had done Peta a disservice as her therapist, neglecting her in a manner similar to so many of her encounters with men. Peta relaxed visibly. She was to tell me many weeks later that this was the first time a man had ever admitted to erring against her and that she had felt empowered since. She had similar arguments with more than one previous male therapist and they had all trivialized her grievances. Therapy has continued to address the issues of mutuality, being heard and having self-needs met within her relationships. Peta and Rowan are no longer a couple.

Discussion

The mistake here concerns myself, as therapist developing my own reputation as an international personality and author, favouring the 'fame' of Rowan, the man, in relation to Peta, the 'invalid' woman. I believe I was engaging with Rowan in an 'I–It' position (we, the famous ones) and excluding Peta, also in an 'I–It' position (you, the undiscovered talent). During this session, Rowan and I had clearly formed 'the Boy's Club' and our male successes were being assessed as far superior to Peta's dormant female potential. Asking Peta for time to contemplate the situation and seek peer supervision, and admitting my error to Peta, appeared to create an opportunity for a different sort of healing relationship. A *meeting* between us evolved in which I *confirmed* my human fallibility and ability to learn and Peta *confirmed* her ability to confront me and let go my past error.

Case 2P: The carpenter

March, 1993: Leonard, 30 years, a carpenter and joiner, complained of the 'wall' that had always been present within his relationships. His last intimacy with Eric, 42, a bank manager, had ended some months earlier. Leonard described Eric as a 'withdrawn' man, very similar to Leonard's alcohol-abusing father, Anthony, who had frequently battered Ruth, Leonard's mother, and had paid little attention to Leonard or his eleven siblings. After our first three meetings, during which I tried to keep the dialogue friendly and 'chatty', Leonard disappeared. He returned two months later and said that he liked me as a therapist but that I talked too much about my own world and that these sessions were his time and *he* wanted to do most of the talking. I expressed my regret that initially I had not heard Leonard accurately, nor tended to his needs sensitively, perhaps in a manner similar to his father and Eric. I had wanted to give Leonard the experience of 'banter' – a conversational realm in which we mutually shared our experiences and in which he would feel safe and empowered. Leonard said that he agreed with my idea of 'banter' but his requirements were to tell his story. Therapy proceeded for a further four months in which I listened to Leonard's dreams, memories and fantasies, largely without interruption. The only input I offered was when Leonard told of a past LSD experience in which he felt he was disintegrating and he had wandered around for days, in a daze, wearing his baseball cap to 'keep his brains in'. I commented: 'Do you think that the LSD took you back to a time when you were very young, perhaps pre-verbal, and you were remembering the sights and sounds of Anthony's abuse of Ruth and your fear and helplessness in this situation?' Leonard smiled and said that the description helped 'name' his experience of disintegration. Leonard said that his wall was disappearing and that he appeared to be taking charge more in his own life and asserting himself within his social network.

Discussion

When I met Leonard, I had in my mind the concept of therapeutic 'banter'(Gunzburg 1993) which has worked so well in so much of the therapy in which I have participated. In preconceiving what might work for Leonard, I missed hearing what he wanted. I believe I held him within an 'I–It' position, a client worthy of the redoubtable Dr Gunzburg's fail-safe banter! Leonard had the courage to assert himself to me, I accommodated my therapeutic style more to what he wanted and we shifted our therapeutic direction. Leonard revealed to me much later that making his needs known to me had been a significant effector of change for him. My assuming what Leonard wanted can be considered as patriarchal: the therapeutic expert determining what is best for the client. My listening to Leonard and entering a therapeutic mode which highlighted his requirements and self-knowledge can be regarded as co-operative; encouraging *meeting, inclusion* and *genuine dialogue.*

Case 2Q: Seeing beneath the surface

June, 1993: Sue, 37 years, a nurse, and her family had seen me over a yearly period. We had discussed how Sue's marriage with Austin, 45, a stockbroker, might be more rewarding and how their son James, 17, might become more motivated towards his schoolwork. Austin himself had seen me previously, on my own, to work on some problems (Gunzburg 1993, pp.353–355). During a joint session with Austin, Sue had told me of some recurring dreams that she had experienced throughout the previous month. I had not responded to Sue's dreams, being more interested to discuss how things were going with the family, and Sue posted me a letter and poem (part of which is reproduced below) the subsequent week.

> Dear Dr. Gunzburg,
>
> What brought me back to see you were the dreams I had been having which were quite clear and vivid. I had begun to feel disturbed by them and since you had been of help to me in the past, I thought you may have been able to help me now before another crisis arose.
>
> You weren't really interested in the dreams except on a superficial level. That is my perception.
>
> My expectations of today's session were that Austin and I would talk about the relationship and that then I would be able to talk about the

real issue of concern to me personally. I think I had a different agenda! Perhaps that's why I felt silly and superfluous at today's session.

The real issue of concern to me is the type of scars left after being used in a sexual way by a trusted adult when I was a child. I find this very difficult to talk about but somehow I am confused as to my reasons and motives for my behaviour and thinking especially in relation to my marriage.

I would like to make an appointment to put this matter to rest because I think it still affects me. I will only make the appointment if you think you can help me as I do not want to waste either your time or my own.

Thank you for your help in the past. It has been very much appreciated.

Yours in good faith,

Sue.

It rained today.
Cold today.
Mozart to brighten
and lighten, today.

She sat, she listened,
wished to be somewhere
else.
Not acknowledged
Not certain
Of trusting the
Stranger who once
offered a helping
hand.

Towards the end
her anger began
to blow
and so
it was quickly
ended.

This session
she expected
to get to the
bottom of her
problem
in relating to those

of the opposite
point of view.

Out she walked
her head held high
but knowing
the thee and thou
were once more
wrapped up
inside.

The soul aches
a little with this
sadness of the
end of things.
Is there no
Turning back?

Can she face
again this other
person and speak
of long ago hurts
that still colour
the way she thinks
and sometimes
acts?

It takes a certain
courage, a certain
kind of strength
and willingness
of others
to see beneath
the surface
tension.

I telephoned Sue, acknowledged my discounting of her dreams during our last meeting and, during a series of individual sessions, Sue started to discuss the painful feelings resulting from her childhood sexual abuse – an event that she had revealed to no one else.

Discussion

Sue's letter and poem brought me to tears. Having seen Sue and her family together previously, I was initially more interested in how the family as a whole was functioning and ignored Sue's introduction of her dreams. Once again I had engaged a client in an 'I–It' position, being more interested in the mode of therapy than the person who had come to see me. Sue signalled to me creatively her discomfort at being disregarded and I immediately acknowledged my participation in discounting her. Sue returned to therapy to discuss an entirely new matter: her sexual abuses in childhood. My original assumption that a family framework was the appropriate one in which to work presumed that my knowledge was more significant than that of the client.

Note the processes of my erring, and healing the breach, that I have tried to illustrate in Cases 2O – 2Q. During the therapeutic process, I engaged in an 'I–It' position with my clients which resulted in my discounting them. This upset our *meeting*, creating an atmosphere of unsafety for my clients and a distance between us. The clients all showed the courage to draw my attention to how they had been ignored and, in each case, I was ready to acknowledge that I had done so. When we resumed therapy, their wisdom was highlighted and they directed the future path of their therapy. But I am left wondering 'what about those clients who were not able to speak out when I discounted them?'

The feminist map

> What a piece of work is a man! How noble in reason! how infinite in faculty! in form and moving, how express and admirable! in action, how like an angel! in apprehension, how like a god! the beauty of the world! the paragon of animals!
>
> (*Hamlet* II.2.323–328)

During a survey in Melbourne in 1993 (The 'Age', June 3rd and 4th), more than 14,000 calls reporting domestic violence were noted – an increase of 26 per cent in a year. An estimated 321,000 people claimed to be direct victims of violence. Thirty-nine per cent of homicides stemmed from domestic conflict. Some people actually considered that domestic violence was permissible in certain circumstances, for example a partner having an affair (15%), a partner refusing to have sex (8%), and a partner failing to fulfill household duties (6%). My belief is that such excuses are unacceptable. Because the majority of my clients are adult survivors of abuse, I pay heed to feminist principles.

Leupnitz writes:

> There are many kinds of feminism. A non-exhaustive list would include liberal, Marxist, Zionist, Christian, radical, and lesbian separatist feminism. What unites them is the desire to reform the social order in ways that would permit the full economic, political, and social participation of women. Feminists believe that gender is socially constituted, not biologically given, and that transformation of those social definitions is possible. Most feminists believe that women and men suffer, although in different ways, from the set of social relationships known as *patriarchy*. Feminism is not a gender. Not all women are feminists and some men are. Feminists disagree about issues such as the origin of women's oppression and, of course, tactics of change. (1988, p.14)

> The word *patriarchy*...also requires explication. If it were not such an important word, one might prefer to leave it out, simply because it has been both misused and misunderstood (1988, p.16). While under earlier forms of patriarchy it was a *male* person who limited the woman's expenditures, freedom to work, and sexual activity in the case of public patriarchy, it is the state, the welfare agency, and the media that control these things (1988, p.17). Ackerman seems to have idealized the mid-nineteenth-century father, writing about him that 'wife and child deferred to his superior wisdom. He exercised his authority firmly but fairly. His discipline was strict but not abusive... Sometimes he became the tyrant; if so, in the end he suffered for the abuse of his power. Echoes of this older image still persist, but they have grown dim (1958, p.179). This portrait is historically inaccurate; To call it a reversal of the facts would not be a gross exaggeration. Wife and child beating were legion in the mid-nineteenth century. The 'tyrant' did not regularly suffer for his tyranny, as there were no laws against beating family members and the culture required female obedience in many ways. (1988, p.32)

Feminist and pro-feminist male therapists believe that the therapeutic conversation should always take into account the historical and present oppression of women.

Along with the many case studies recorded in this book, I share the following stories with clients when inviting them to consider issues concerning patriarchy.

Case 2R: Beating the odds[11]

June, 1993: Jane, a journalist, currently receiving the invalid pension, was dejected about her future. She had an extremely poor opinion of men, and not without good reason. She had witnessed her father, an abuser of alcohol, ignore and discount her mother throughout her childhood. The mother had expressed her frustration through over-zealous discipline of her four children. The only way for Jane's mother to get the father's attention appeared to be to scream! Jane was certain that both parents genuinely cared for the material welfare of their children, but there seemed to have been no softness or affirmation. The father prevented Jane's mother, a former saleswoman, from pursuing a career. Secretly, the mother had studied and completed several secondary school subjects. Ten years previously, Jane had divorced Keith, a graphic designer, after six years marriage. Keith had contributed neither income nor emotional support for Jane, or their off-spring, and seemed to have relied on Jane for his every need. Moreover, Keith also resisted Jane's continuing education – in a similar manner to her father. Keith said that he was not going to be coerced into working for a living and ignored Jane's pleas for support. She had become depressed and 'crazy with the stress of having to do it all' and had left the family. After a two-year custody battle, during which there was joint access of their children, Jane had yielded custody to Keith and his new partner. Jane felt that, had she remained, she would have developed into a frustrated disciplinarian like her mother and she did not want that experience for her children. Though Jane communicated regularly with them, she was still grieving and felt guilty over the distance that she had established between herself and them. Jane then met Davy, a labourer, who proved to be a violent heroin addict and she left him three years later after experiencing an early end to two pregnancies; one being terminated, the other being ectopic.

Two years later, whilst travelling overseas, Jane conceived during a friendship with a man well-known within his own country. When interviewed regarding termination of the pregnancy, the hospital doctor had proven courteous and compassionate but, when he heard that the father was from his own culture, the doctor became very critical and performed surgery without any anaesthetic. Not only was this excruciatingly painful, it was a dangerous practice, exposing Jane to the significant risk of post-operative shock. Since that time, Jane had suffered loss of energy and was unable to work. Her poor concentration interfered with her creativity and she experienced constant neck and shoulder spasms.

---

11 This case was originally presented in the 'General Practitioner', *Adis International 2*, 1, January 1993, 9.

I felt outraged! 'It sounds as if that doctor was punishing you for a misdemeanour, breaking the rules of his community. Yours is a story of real torture. I am dismayed to hear it'. Jane burst into tears and said that she had told no one about this event until that moment.

Our conversation continued. We discussed whether Jane had been punishing herself by having a succession of pregnancies to replace her 'lost' children and then terminating them because of her feelings of unworthiness. If she was punishing herself, was it a life sentence? Was there no Court of Appeal? In fact, might not her action in leaving her children when she did be considered a form of 'loving', sparing them from the oppressive parenting that she might have duplicated from her mother? Their father had assumed a responsible role at that time and now that they appeared to be growing into adolescence without too much fuss, wasn't it time to consider the most rewarding future relationship that she might enjoy with them: to recover her health and participate within life in a different and refreshing manner?

We discussed the film *Raise the Red Lantern*, concerning the apparent options open to women in a strictly patriarchal society: to be sad, and perhaps suicide? to be bad, and be punished? or to become mad, and end up isolated? We considered how Jane's male partners had relegated responsibility for birth control to her and how her father and Keith had both hindered their female partners' career paths. Would the women have behaved differently if they had not been so obstructed? We queried why Keith had taken such a lengthy time to assume responsibility for their children.

Jane had been struggling, unsuccessfully, for months to obtain funding for a vocational retraining programme. The employment officer's attitude seemed to have been: 'Is that *really* an appropriate job for you to seek?' Jane has decided to stop pursuing work through that avenue, has obtained a student loan and organized a writer's clinic to pay for it at the end of the year. Her energy levels are steadily increasing and she maintains contact with her teenagers. Jane appears to be beating the odds!

Discussion

Jane's, and her mother's, actions suggested that they had slipped into the traditional patriarchal role of being 'carer' to their men. Feminism would regard patriarchal culture as placing men and women within an 'I–It' position, individuals being subservient to the roles placed on them. Within such roles, there can be no *meeting* or *genuine dialogue* between the genders, nor can women and minors be *included* within the patriarch's experience.

Women and minors remain mere extensions of the patriarch's experience. Jane's father, Keith and Davy all acted as though their needs were predominant. They criticized and disciplined their women when they perceived them to be making mistakes. Both Jane's father and Keith behaved as if the mother's and Jane's sole duty was to support them and to raise the children. The father and Keith both objected to, and impeded, their female partners following their own careers. Jane became overwhelmed over a lengthy period of time, leading to her leaving the family and losing custody of her children. She suffered feelings that only 'bad mothers deserted their children' and 'bad mothers deserved to lose their children'. Both Jane and her mother appeared to have used two ploys permitted to women to get their needs met in a patriarchal community: Jane's mother had become 'mad' with anger, screaming at her husband and children, and Jane had become 'sad', developing depression. At the risk of appearing tedious, I have stressed these issues concerning patriarchy repeatedly because they occur so frequently in the families of origin, and current families, of survivors of abuse. What is as horrifying in Jane's story is the extent of institutional abuse: the doctor who 'punished' her affair with a member of his ethnic group by operating on her without anaesthetic and the dictatorial attitudes of the petty bureaucrat to Jane's initiative for pursuing a vocation. Perhaps these institutional violations are related to the most significant question that many contemporary therapists are asking: we may be able to facilitate survivors of violence in their empowerment, and encourage their abusers to take responsibility for their violations, but how do we invite those people in politics, business, the legal and medical professions, the media and academic circles (these institutions still being largely dominated by men) to take seriously the influence of patriarchy on violent behaviours within the community?

Case 2S: The property manager

July, 1992: Joyce, 39 years, a property manager, was distressed at her inability to end her relationship with her lover of thirteen years, Don, 45, unemployed and bankrupt. Don and Joyce had experienced an 'on again, off again' relationship, with Don always leaving to go and live with his wife, Carol, 41, an accountant, and three young adult children. Joyce said that whenever Don lived with her, he told her that he could not stand the guilt that he had betrayed his family and he would return 'repentant' to them again. Don had financially impoverished the family with his instability and indecision and said that they, indeed all his relatives, now hated him with a passion. Six years before, when Don lay in an intensive care ward with severe head injuries, Joyce and Carol arrived at the hospital at the same time and the nursing staff were confused. Both women obviously knew Don intimately and both had been registered as his wife in their records! Joyce's family had also 'given up' on her, not wanting to know anything more of her relationship with Don. Joyce did not know what to do. She said that there were many warm moments with Don. He appeared to be compassionate, warm and loving, then would disappear without explanation. Joyce said that she had wanted to end the relationship many times in the past few years but Don would always find a way to intrude into her territory again. She had changed the locks to her home, but he had broken in. She had put out a restraining order on him, but he had ignored it, coming to her workplace and pleading with Joyce to take him back. Quite recently, Don had approached Joyce in a car park of a supermarket and she had attacked him in a rage. I asked Joyce if she would write Don a letter of goodbye. Joyce wrote:

Dear Don,

This probably is the most difficult letter I have ever had to write. I had hoped that by replying to your last letter and stating that I 'honestly' did not want you to pursue me, you would have taken me at my word, but your visit to my office Saturday morning proved that, as usual, you took no notice of my decision that the relationship is over.

There is nothing more to be gained by writing of my anger toward you, or the hurt I feel. We have been over and over that ground so many times it has become like a broken record. I am still experiencing those feelings, together with a kind of grief. I am mourning the loss of you and the loss of a relationship I gave my whole being to make work, but my whole being was not enough. Perhaps I gave too much, you often told me so.

For me, all that remains now is to pick up the pieces, to regain my self-esteem and to build a new life for myself, by myself. I thank you for the good times we shared and there were many. Hopefully, in time, it will be the good things that spring to mind when I think of you and the rest will fade away. To be honest, I can't blame you entirely. It was my choice to keep taking you back, to believe each time that this time would be different, that you really meant what you said. I wanted to believe it, and each time I filed away all the pain from the time before. I put the pain to the back of my mind but I could never lose the mistrust. My inability to believe you, my need to double check and ultimately, each time, to find that my doubts were justified, had distorted my personality and changed me into someone I have little respect for.

It's time for me to move on Don. I want to feel good about myself, to be confident and self-assured. I don't want to constantly be looking over my shoulder waiting for the next bolt of lightening to knock me down and find myself becoming weaker with each strike.

You have always admired my strength, that has always been part of your attraction to me. I know that I can never regain that strength until I make the final break with you.

I wish you luck and happiness and I sincerely hope you wish the same for me. Please let this be the end.

Joyce posted this letter. Don's response was to turn up unexpectedly to a session of therapy. Joyce invited him in. Don was adamant that he and Joyce could make a go of it, even at this late stage. He appeared completely unaware how, through his actions, he had been unable to contribute a measure of safety to either his family or to Joyce. I continued to see Joyce weekly. 'You are probably going to throw me out of your room', Joyce said one day, 'but Don's back living with me. Don showed me the papers seeking divorce from Carol that he had his lawyer prepare. He has never done that before. I shall give Don another go, but take it day-by-day, not expecting too much'. After four more sessions, Joyce said: 'He's gone. I found out that he had rescinded the divorce papers the day before they were to go through. He just packed his bags and left. I have sent the remainder of his belongings to his daughter's house'. Joyce and I commenced working on ways to fortify her boundaries: assertive phrases, legal action and police protection from harassment, in case Don wishes to 'conciliate'. Joyce expressed her feelings of foolishness that she had taken so long to make a decision to be rid of Don. We shared the image of Don very much like the Tyrannosaurus rex in Steven Spielberg's film *Jurassic Park* – lumbering, predatory, relentless, not immediately knowing which car contained the tastier meal (the one with the adults or the one with the children). The words, as I remembered them, of a character from Nora Ephron's bitter-sweet comedy-drama *Heartburn* also came to mind. The wife, played by Meryl Streep, has discovered yet again that her husband, played by Jack Nicholson, has been philandering – as he has done so many times during their marriage. Just before she throws the lemon meringue pie in the husband's face, the wife exclaims: 'Why do we stay with them when we know that they're cheating on us? We are not stupid. Why do we stay? We stay with them because we hope they will change!'.

Three months after Don had left, Joyce handed me the following document:

My retirement from a crisis lifestyle

In retrospect, very few of my 39 years have been free of the crisis lifestyle. The early crises in my life were not of my own doing, but happened with such regularity that I accepted the patterns as normal. I didn't realise then, in fact have never realised until now, that by normalising that pattern, it became habit, an addiction. I had no will to break free. I accepted the ongoing crises as unavoidable, inevitable. I hoped that if I could hold on a little longer, surely paradise would appear. It didn't.

Somewhere along the line I lost the instinct, if indeed I ever had it, to know when enough is enough. Hanging in there for the good while trying to overlook the bad can never work. Instead of being rewarded in the long run with hope and happiness, it brings trauma, fear and exhaustion. There is no rest.

There is pain in making the break but it gives hope. I can recover. I am ready to do battle. I will no longer accept bad in hope of good. I will not accept less than my worth. I will rebuild my inner self. With a little help, I will memorise the traps and how they were laid. I will live freely instead of falsely.

I have a lot of hard work ahead but the hardest part was to begin. It scares me. I know nothing of this person I am about to discover. She has been hidden deep inside me for such a long, long time, but, at the same time, I am excited, anticipatory, ready to let go of the half-life I have lived until now and to discover a full life. Life begins at 40.

Two years later, Joyce has referred one of her friends to me for some help. The friend says that Joyce soon finished with Don after she completed therapy, has found a pleasant companion and could not be happier!

Discussion

Joyce put a great deal of time and effort in trying to *meet* Don and enter into a *genuine dialogue* with him, 'hoping that he would change'. Don appeared to be holding both women, and his children, within an 'I–It' position, following a romantic script with wife and lover both, and seemingly oblivious to Joyce and/or his family's needs for security and stability. I often comment to people entangled within love triangles, and trying to escape, that the great romantic operas by Verdi, Puccini and Bizet usually end with dead bodies littered all over the stage. Joyce *confirmed* herself as a courageous freedom fighter, willing to face the pain of loss as she broke away from Don. In her retirement from a 'crisis lifestyle', Joyce envisioned a struggle towards an opportunity in which she could regain her self-respect and integrity.

The holistic map

Participating in a therapeutic conversation often utilizes a different mode of thinking from the everyday social encounter; consider the mathematical problem presented in Figure 2.1:[12,13]

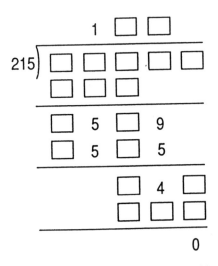

Figure 2.1 The holistic map illustrated by a mathematical problem

To solve this puzzle not only requires knowledge of the rules of long division, but an ability to stand back, consider the spaces, conceptualize what is missing and discover what is needed to complete the pattern. Participating within the therapeutic conversation is not dissimilar. It demands cognizance of many therapeutic frameworks (some of which have been introduced in this section) and, also, a capacity in therapists to 'step outside' their interactions with clients, view their encounters holistically and ascertain what needs to be done to invite clients to change.

---

12   The answer to this puzzle is 37195 divided by 215 equals 173
13   This figure was originally presented in Gunzburg 1991, p.13.

I share the following stories with clients when inviting them to consider that we may discover together another angle from which to view their struggles – one which offers resolution or, at least, a less difficult direction in the future.

Case 2T: Scoring[14]

It was May 1983 and Myra, 61 years, was experiencing yet another dose of 'the guilts'. Born to an authoritarian, religious family, she had divorced her husband two decades earlier. Divorce had been against the dogma of her religion and Myra had tormented herself about her 'bad faith' ever since. Even worse, she had compounded her wickedness by entering into a relationship with Gordon, 55, a widower, whom Myra liked and respected very much. There was none of the negativity and isolation that Myra had experienced during her previous marriage.

'Yes, doctor, I am having sex with him', Myra had answered unasked, 'and no, doctor, we have no future plans for a wedding'. Myra really did enjoy the physical side of the friendship but could not accept that it was all out of wedlock. 'I feel like a slut', she muttered. 'I should know when to leave it alone'. As I listened to Myra, I quietly drifted off into a trance state for a few minutes and found myself fantasizing: I was playing electronic video games and becoming very frustrated because I was not achieving really high scores. 'You really have very high expectations of yourself, don't you?', I commented suddenly, with an unusual abruptness that surprised myself. 'A bit of a perfectionist, aren't you?'. Myra sat up just as abruptly and ceased her stream of self-deprecation. 'I had never thought of it like that before', she responded.

Our conversation turned to the high expectations Myra's parents had held for her. She felt that she had tried so very hard – at school, within her marriage – to please them and had never been able to achieve this. Over the next few therapy sessions (Myra attended weekly) we were able to discuss how Myra was projecting her parent's high expectations onto her concept of God, regarding her God as one who demanded the impossible standards of her parents (e.g. perpetuation of a lifeless and unrewarding marriage, rigid roles and denial of life unless certain forms were observed – such as intimacy only within the marriage contract). Myra ended therapy after fourteen months, blaming herself hardly at all, and with obvious improvement in the enjoyment of her partnership with Gordon. It had become a gilt-edged experience, rather than a guilt-edged one.

---

14 This case was originally presented in *Patient Management 14,* 12, December 1990, 43–8.

Discussion

Myra appeared to be concentrating on the 'sinful aspects' of her personal behaviour. In labelling her actions as 'badness, weakness, irresponsible and undisciplined, all worthy of punishment, Myra seemed to be viewing herself within an I–It position. I believe therapy was effective by:

1. Initially inviting Myra into a therapeutic conversation without expecting too much change. The first months were spent rather quietly as Myra told me her story without my making undue demands on her to perform. I believe it was during this phase that *meeting* between Myra and myself occurred.

2. Taking time out to let my unconscious mind play with the information being received. This is an excellent example of *imagining the real*: the high scores of the fantasized computer games reflecting Myra's high expectations of herself. I was able to tune into an important theme in Myra's life: the quest for perfection. This can be regarded as a missing piece of the puzzle in Myra's struggle. She had learnt to live up to the high expectations of her family of origin and was not aware that she was making these same unreasonable demands on herself in her current life.

3. Making overt this theme to Myra: how she was living up to the expectations of others, including her God. My abruptness startled me and I feared, momentarily, that I had been too spontaneous and challenging. However, Myra very rapidly stopped her self-criticism and appeared to accept my invitation to consider another world-view: she was not inherently 'evil', rather she had been taught by her parents to strive unrelentingly towards unreasonable goals. When she failed to achieve these goals, she felt powerless and disesteemed. I believe that this was one point at which Myra and I experienced mutual *inclusion* within our experiencing of the world, when we reached an I–Thou position. Most of us find ourselves struggling at some time against unrealistic expectations and here we were, joint participants in a therapeutic conversation about this issue.

4. Discussing how life could be different: Did God demand impossible standards, rigid roles, lack of autonomy and initiative or denial of sexual intimacy where respect and liking was present between partners? Such a deity would surely view people within an I–It

position. Instead, I invited Myra to contemplate a God with whom she could enjoy an I–Thou intimacy, one who allowed responsibility, concern and pleasure in life, rather than a limiting adherence to 'the right way'. Myra was, I believe, more able to examine her attitudes and choices, to change and *confirm* herself.

Case 2U: A dying angel[15]

July, 1988: Cliff, 18 years, was telling me of the anxiety attacks that had been plaguing him for the past eighteen months. He was at the point of commencing a promising career as a concert pianist and the feedback as to his future direction had been most encouraging. We talked for a while about the musical tradition in his family. Cliff's grandmother, apparently, had shown great talent as a pianist but had put aside career opportunities to raise a family. Her daughter, Cliff's mother, was an orchestral cellist. Cliff's father was an orchestral viola player who had always wanted to be a virtuoso violinist. I remarked how the music seemed to have gained greater expression through the generations and wondered if Cliff experienced this as a pressure, a family expectation to succeed. Cliff said that he did not. I asked Cliff what his favourite piece of music was. Cliff nominated the Berg violin concerto: 'It expresses so much turbulence during the earlier movements, then resolves itself so peacefully. Berg was married to Mahler's daughter, you know. He dedicated this concerto to another of Mahler's daughters, who had died prematurely. Berg called the concerto "Death of an Angel"'. 'And an angel is dying in your life also', I added quietly. Cliff's mother had been diagnosed as having a malignant breast tumour eighteen months previously. There were tears and sadness, and we discussed what Cliff would like to achieve in the relationship with his mother during the time that was left to them. Cliff's anxiety attacks disappeared.

Discussion

I endeavoured to highlight the following themes that were weaving through the therapeutic conversation and invited Cliff to consider which of these were missing pieces of the puzzle behind his anxiety attacks:

1. The normal stresses in the life of a young person entering a new and demanding career.

2. The possible pressures of a family musical tradition on Cliff (i.e. the need to 'perpetuate the faith' and to excel).

---

15 This case was originally presented in *Patient Management 14*, 12, December 1990, 43–8.

3. The effect of the mother's terminal illness on Cliff.

This last may have created the most impact, leading to our *meeting* and *including* us both in a *genuine dialogue* about the universal theme of loss, and resulting in Cliff grieving with tears rather than panic.

I had seen Cliff's mother, Rebecca, 52, for two to three sessions of therapy before her son had actually attended. She had been very depressed as to her cancer and I had asked her to compose a piece of music or write a song to be performed at her funeral. The lift in Rebecca's mood at the next therapy session had been quite remarkable. The missing pieces of the puzzle behind Rebecca's depression may be brought into focus in the form of questions: how to be productive in the time left? how to battle against all odds? how to cheat death? how can creativity arise out of decay? how can Rebecca give towards the future? Rebecca was a Jewish woman who had lived largely outside her religion; creativity had been her creed. Now, in her decline, she described feelings of warmth, nostalgia and yearning for those Jewish origins long past, and we discussed the possibilities of a Jewish funeral. The missing pieces of the puzzle here may be found in further queries: how can Rebecca return to her group? how can she achieve belonging and permanence?

As Rebecca left my room, she turned to me and said: 'I do hope that I have not mollycoddled Cliff and doted on him too much as he has grown up. I do not want to find him too dependent on "my having been there" for him, after I have died'. 'Madam', I replied, 'just because Freud loved his mother and feared his father does not mean that every good Jewish boy has to do the same!' There were smiles from us both.

Case 2V: The cellist[16]

March, 1987: Sally, a 25 years, an art teacher, was concerned that her boyfriend, Ben, 26, was becoming unbalanced. They had had a relationship for the past two-and-a-half years and, for the last six months, had been quarrelling constantly. Moreover, Ben was drinking more alcohol than usual, was driving erratically and had mentioned that a former friend, Doug, had strange and powerful influences over him. Ben had talked of 'doing away with Doug' to break his evil hold. It certainly sounded as if Ben was heading for a psychotic breakdown – the symptoms for which anti-schizophrenic medication might be recommended – and I invited Sally to bring Ben with her to a subsequent session.

When next seen a week later, Sally arrived early and stated that Ben had told her that he would come to this session but, if there was any 'bad-mouth-

16 This case was originally presented in Gunzburg 1991, pp.217–8.

ing' of him, he would leave. Ben arrived five minutes later and proceeded to tell me of his hopes and dreams. He was an orchestral cellist, well-known throughout Australia, and had been advised that he had the potential to attain international renown. The troubles between Sally and himself had erupted when he had begun to practise his instrument seriously, with the idea that he would pursue a solo career, six months previously. Ben had agonized over the demands that would be made on Sally as the wife of a virtuoso: many months a year spent apart on tour, with little support for Sally's own vocational and personal growth as she would be channelling her efforts into caring for what family they might have. Perhaps, some years hence, when he was more certain of his own direction, he would select a mate. Ben had spent the past few days drinking whisky in an effort to relieve his distress.

I praised Ben for being so clear about his wishes and concern for Sally. I commented that it appeared that this couple's problems had started when Ben had made a definite decision to divert his attention, six months earlier, towards his career goals. It seemed a pity, if he had the talent and skills, not to develop them. Sally's choice appeared to be deciding whether she wanted to play the role required of her or not. With a look of relief, Sally replied that she had been troubled about Ben's career also and that she did not really want to be a celebrity's spouse. The two left my room amicably with Sally requesting a couple more sessions to ventilate her feelings of loss that Ben, at this stage, did not wish to add another string to his bow.

Discussion

Sally presented her boyfriend's erratic behaviour in terms of whether he was 'going mad or not'. Sally appeared to view Ben within an I–It position and there is a temptation, especially for medically-trained therapists, to join Sally in this framework and diagnose Ben with a mental illness. Rather, Ben, Sally and I joined in a *meeting* and listened to Ben's story. I invited Ben and Sally to consider Ben's reactions in terms of Ben facing a transitional crisis in his life: whether to settle with Sally into a permanent relationship or to follow a promising career. Ben indicated that he had thought about the consequences of his decision ethically and responsibly. The drinking, rather than being delinquent behaviour, could be considered a way to lessen his stress. This can be regarded as the missing piece of the puzzle: Ben's 'madness' being part of his struggle to effect an equitable outcome for Sally and himself. Sally found that she too had choices to make. Asking Ben and Sally both to consider their dilemmas *included* all of us within the therapeutic conversation. We all have to make choices for our own needs, impinging on the needs of our intimates some of the time. Ben and Sally appeared to be able to resolve their problem when viewing it within the context of a human interactional drama rather than an expression of Ben's mental dissolution. I believe that they were able to *confirm* themselves as people able to make choices towards their own independence and growth whilst, at the same time, being able to negotiate a respectful separation, choices and negotiations made within an I–Thou position.

Case 2W: Crucified[17]

August, 1985: I was observing Renata, 32 years, working with Felicia, 43, a divorcee, and her two children, Briony, 14, and Morton, 12, at the family therapy centre where we both worked. I was watching Renata and the family via closed-circuit television in an adjacent room. Renata was sitting opposite Felicia with Briony seated on her right and Morton placed on her left. They were discussing issues of discipline (Morton and Briony would not participate in family routines without a great deal of fuss) and every time Felicia and Renata came close to the crux of the problem and looked like reaching solutions, Briony and/or Morton would interject and interrupt the dialogue. Half-way through the session, Renata left the family and took a break to bounce some ideas about family process off me. 'Look at the way you are all seated', I said, 'in a crucifix pattern. I wonder if Felicia perceives you as the family's saviour?' 'Funny you should say that', Renata commented. 'Felicia has rung me three times this week to ask me for advice'.

When Renata rejoined the family, she sat next to Felicia and positioned Briony and Morton next to each other. By the session's end, Renata had been able to encourage the children to commence negotiating dishwashing rosters, privacy in bedrooms and choice of television programmes with each other.

Discussion

In inviting Renata to consider the crucifix seating arrangement of this family, I can be regarded as offering her a missing piece of the puzzle. This family appeared to be viewing Renata within an I–It position: you are our saviour who will save us from further distress. Altering the seating patterns can be considered as *including* family members and Renata in a different arrangement:

- It allied the two adults, enabling Renata to model parenting techniques more effectively. This *confirmed* Renata's role as therapist.

---

17 This case was originally presented in *Patient Management 14*, 12, December 1990, 43–8.

○ it enabled Briony and Morton to interact more capably within the sibling sub-system. This *confirmed* their role as siblings.

The spiritual map

People often regard themselves as embroiled in a battle of their wills against the harsh vissicitudes of life. Life is Nature, and Nature doesn't give a damn! or, as Buber might have said, many people believe that Life always views them within an I–It position. The therapeutic conversation encourages the healing of its participants by inviting them to be *included* within a wider, cohesive, nourishing and disciplined communal group. Participants can divert their preoccupation with their 'struggling self' towards a concept of mutually interrelated individuals and become *confirmed* by integrating within a wider system that is 'the good' or God.

Case 2X: The touch[18]

July, 1988: Gary's general practitioner asked me if I could see his patient that day as he appeared to be severely depressed and suicide could be a very real outcome.

For about thirty minutes, Gary, 47 years, sat in my room withdrawn and non-communicative, with a downcast mien. Then he revealed that he was employed as a printer and had also developed skills as a landscape artist. He had ceased attending work a week previously because he could cope no longer and it had been months since he had attempted painting. His mother, in New Zealand, was dying. 'I should be there for her', Gary asserted, 'and I cannot get time off to see her until Christmas (six months away). I should be there for her now! – she was there for me when I was comatose after a car accident during my teens'. I leaned forward and, gently resting a hand on Gary's shoulder, responded: 'It must be very difficult for you being here, with your mother, who has been so devoted to you, over there – you cannot even reach out to her.'

Gary returned three days later, bright as a button. He had returned to work, was negotiating early leave of absence with his boss to visit New Zealand and had taken up his brush again. We chatted about Gary's artistry – how he painted while listening to varied pieces of music which matched his mood; how he had to stand back from a scene, tear the pieces apart internally, then reconstruct them attuned to his own unique character and express them on canvas for observers who could then connect the completed picture with their own internal experience.

---

18 This case was originally presented in *Patient Management 13*, 1, January 1989, 65–8.

Discussion

All of Buber's ideas can be considered to weave within this example of fairly simple, though not simplistic, therapeutic conversation:

- Being with clients and not pushing too hard for a response; letting clients know that their needs for privacy are respected. Therapists and clients can indeed *meet* each other during silence.

- Gently offering an opportunity for conversation, inviting clients to participate within a *genuine dialogue.*

- Hearing clients' messages clearly, that is 'I feel guilty – my mother, who cared for me, needs me and I'm not there'. In hearing Gary's message clearly, I was able to *imagine the real* experience from Gary's perspective: his loneliness, anxiety and frustration. Often clients come to therapy viewing their problems within an I–It position, that is when Gary says 'I should be there for her', he can be considered as speaking within an I–It position, 'I should be there for her, I should be doing better than I am, I am a "bad" son, I am an "It", filled with badness'. The therapeutic conversation aims to place the clients' feelings and actions within a different context. It invites clients to shift from an I–It position to an I–Thou position, one in which they are included within the struggles and strengths of the wider community.

- Reacting in an appropriate way to let clients know that they are understood, that is 'You want to reach out to your mother (accompanied by me touching Gary's shoulder) and you cannot'. Reaching out and touching Gary, at that particular moment, can be regarded as an act of mutual *inclusion*; the compassionate therapist comforting the distressed client. We all need to be comforted and comforters at various stages of our life. Through this action, Gary and I can be considered as becoming mutually interrelated.

- Conversing within Gary's perspective and matching it with the interactional processes occurring within the therapy room – the artistry of taking pieces of human experience apart, reorganizing them and recreating them into a more effective whole – can be considered a conversation during which both therapists and clients connect with each other within an I–Thou position. Within the I–Thou position, therapists and clients can *confirm* each other as whole spiritual beings. The I–Thou position can be viewed as the quintessential spiritual position in which therapists and clients, and their perspectives, are included within the whole communal network, through their conversation, through their creativity, through their good-will...

Case 2Y: A ray of hope

In November 1992, Ray, 34 years, administrator of an electrical retail firm, told me of his depression and fear of failure that had been present since primary school. Over a few weekly sessions of therapy, Ray described his religiously fundamentalist, authoritarian father, Paul, 68, who had breathed the terror of God into Ray if he did not do his best and had administered strict punishments if Ray failed to meet the father's expectations. Ray said that he had been timid and hesitant to take risks ever since leaving home. Nonetheless, Ray had married Janine, 37, a secretary, eighteen months previously and was enjoying their four-month-old son, Joshua and David and Sharon, Janine's children by a previous marriage. Deeply religious himself, Ray said that it had been many years since he had prayed in any substantial manner to God and, though work and family routines were fairly rewarding, he was despairing about finding any emotional fulfillment in his life. I asked Ray if he would compose a prayer to God now. Ray returned to our next session with the suicide note that he had written!:

> By the time you finish reading this communication, my life will be extinguished. Even though I know I have no right contemplating taking my own life at this point in time, it seems the most viable solution. My regrets in this however is the pain it will cause to all I know, especially my family, but probably no more pain than I have caused in life. I hope I can be forgiven in death. I do not seem to fit in anywhere. My life seems to be one of conflict. I have made many mistakes. There is much pain in my physical body. It is all messed up, like a cancer eating away at the foundations of life. My mind can no longer fathom. My spirit is so troubled it has lost its way. My heart has great love and much to give, yet is empty as well. There is much to live for, a future which has great potential and new beginnings. There is my family – Janine, a beautiful woman, the only woman I have ever loved, but unbending, and our son Joshua, born out of love. It is sad his father has come to this end and he will miss me, but maybe someone better will step into the shoes I will leave. There is also David, my step-son, who I consider as my son too (you are not to blame) and Sharon, my step-daughter. I can see no future in my current situation. Financially, it is extremely difficult and I see no improvement. On a

single wage I can never get ahead, even hardly make ends meet. My wage is good, but not great. Relying on the Social Security arena allows me no freedom, and although it is a help, it is also a hindrance. I can never really make that little bit extra. I have let my family down financially. My mistake financially was not saving. Everything was for the here and now and making up for what I never had as I grew up prior to my marriage. My time with the Church saw me give away what I probably should have looked to the future for. Now I have nothing. Parents are unable to help either. I cannot achieve what is needed and see no light here either. The frustration is monumental. On a personal level, I love as much as my heart is capable of loving, but my freedom to love is a prison. It needs to be let out and gently nurtured back into life, but I feel it could be too late now. I have achieved nothing in this life (except Joshua). Nowhere have I left a mark except anguish. My not being part of life will probably make no difference. I guess I really haven't done much and would like to do more, like travel, carry out a hobby, enjoy interests, have a great family life, as much as is or would be possible, live in our own place. I guess I could make a huge list, but…what does it matter? I know that I (we) are better off than most and not as well off as some, but in my own sphere it doesn't seem to count. Most of what I once believed, I no longer hold. Where is my faith? Everything I do, I do for others, and do nothing for myself. I have lost self. Goodbye, I love you all, even though you will probably wish you never knew me. I hope some day, somehow, you may all forgive me as I hope God can forgive me. For God can only save me now, as the night closes in. Who loves me and will let me know? If there is a Heaven, and God forgives me, as I ask His forgiveness, I will look after you all, I promise. Please make the most of what you can in life, and try not to let my action unbalance you too much. I'm sorry. I really do love you all. I just didn't love myself. I have allowed myself to become what I'm not and let go of who I am. I have no identity. What I know is right, I do not do, and I agree too much with what is wrong. For the most part, I have a conscience, others do not seem to.

I discussed with Ray the prayers that seemed to be weaving throughout the text of his letter: give me the freedom to love, grant me a love of self, give me the ability to forgive myself. I commented that, although at the depths of despair, Ray had chosen not to kill himself…perhaps beneath it all there was a Ray of hope! We talked also about whether Ray was trying to fulfill a patriarchal script written for him by his father: men must do their best.

Ray's father had trained him to win at everything, yet Ray appeared to be a very different man from his tyrannical caretaker: kind, gentle, sensitive to Janine and the children. Perhaps Ray was winning at not being like his father? Might not Ray turn some of his kindness towards others towards himself, letting himself 'off the hook' and not continue to 'beat himself up'? Over the next few sessions, Ray's despondency lifted and he started taking the initiative, inviting the family out to a surprise dinner, inviting Janine to be lovers one evening and taking time out to refresh himself in a new hobby.

Discussion

Ray's letter enabled me to *imagine the real* depths of his despair, yearning for a mortal end to his pain, yet also hoping for a freedom to be a whole being once more. Ray's letter facilitated our *meeting*, enabling me to highlight the positive aspects, the prayer in his cry for release. Describing Ray as a battler against patriarchy helps to *confirm* him as a different man from his authoritarian father.

Case 2Z: Redemption[19]

May, 1989: During one of her final sessions, Alma, 40 years, incest survivor, former prostitute and member of Alcoholics Anonymous, arrived wearing spotless white jeans and long-sleeved white shirt. It was the week prior to Yom Kippur, the Day of Atonement, and I shared with Alma how many Jews on this day wore items of white, sometimes being completely clothed in white, to indicate their belief in a new future. We discussed the symbols of salvation in Alma's Catholic faith: Mary and Jesus often pictured in white, as are the Angels, and inevitably our conversation moved on to the After-life.

'I think that y'become part of a spiritual whole, as long as y're kind and decent', remarked Alma. 'What do y'think?'

'I have this belief', I replied, 'that at the moment of my death, the love of all the people I have ever known will flood into me and I will carry this love with me forever. Because I will have no eyes or ears to measure with, the passing of time will not be a bother to me. There is a lot of love, a lot of people there...and you are one of them'. Alma beamed and replied: 'You too!'

Discussion

Alma and I both believed in hope for the future. This belief enabled us to meet and be participants within the therapeutic conversation. I invited Alma

---

19 This case was originally presented in the *Newsletter of the Australian Society of Logotherapy 3*, 2, July 1990, 6–11.

to join with me in Buber's approach of *imagining the real*: taking what is nourishing and useful from both Jewish and Catholic perspectives and synthesizing these values (redemption, positive change, optimism) using the symbol 'white'. We were able to cross-fertilize each other's views and strengthen our personal values and, in so doing, *confirm* ourselves. In sharing our thoughts on 'life after death', we *included* ourselves within each other's world-view. This belief of the After-life is entrenched in both our religions and both of us had adapted it to our own unique needs. We found that our beliefs connected finite and infinite, the specific with the universal and ourselves with each other. Therapeutic love proved a great redeemer for us both!

This story very much illustrates my belief in exploring how people limit themselves in the beliefs that they bring with them into the therapy room (beliefs that are usually grounded within an I–It position) and in encouraging a system of values that enriches life, rather than diminishes it (a system which includes client and therapist with the rest of the community within an I–Thou position). If we must believe, then we might as well believe in something that is useful, in values that we ourselves have experienced as rewarding, that help us to esteem ourselves. As Buber would have it: 'values are not determined objectively by a body outside of ourselves, by dealing in abstract ideas, theories and notions. Values are discovered experientially within the encounter of persons meeting in goodwill, within the life of dialogue' (Friedman 1960, p.278). My belief is that the therapeutic conversation is such an encounter.

> Jaacob Yitzchak reflected as he contemplated symbols cut into the ancient table in front of his seat, symbols which apparently formed the initials of his names. Then he began. 'My first story will be called: "How I Apprenticed Myself to a Smith." When I was boarding in Apt in the house of my father-in-law, the baker, the window of my room looked out on a smithy. When I would take my seat at my window in the morning with my book, the fire of the smithy was already blazing and the bellows hissed and the smith, almost without taking a breath, beat down on the anvil. The ringing of the hammer on the anvil was the accompaniment of my daily morning studies. But as time went on I could no longer bear to find the man already at work before I had begun. I arose somewhat earlier. It availed nothing. The hammering over there was in full blast and the sparks flew to the very street. I got up still earlier; it still availed nothing. 'I cannot let that mere mechanic put me to shame – me who am striving after the life eternal,' I said to myself and sought again to get the better of him. In vain. Thus things

went on for awhile, until I arose so early that I had to light a candle to read my book. It was too strange to endure any longer. I went downstairs and entered the smithy. The man ceased working at once and asked after my desire. I told him of the experience I had had with him and begged him to tell me when he began to work. 'Until a short time ago,' he answered, 'I began at the usual hour. We smiths are all early risers. But then I saw that every day a little later than I you came to the window and began to read. Thereupon I said to myself that I could not very well permit someone who strains nothing but his head to offer me competition. So I went to my anvil earlier and earlier. Yet it availed me nothing, for always you were already there.' 'You cannot possibly understand,' I said to him, 'what I have at stake in my work.' 'Undoubtedly I cannot,' he replied, 'but can you understand what I have at stake in mine?' Thus I learned that it is necessary to understand what our fellows have at stake.

'Oho,' cried one of the students, who had been growling to himself for some time. 'You are evidently one of those who would like to understand everybody and everything!' 'Not at all,' Jaacob Yitzchak replied. 'But since that experience it strikes me unseemly to question another's understanding of me, while I have not yet come to understand him.' (Buber 1981, pp.30–1)

Section Three

If you want to help someone out of the mire, be prepared to get
yourself a little dirty. (The Baal Shem, Buber 1947, p.7)

Creating tales of empowerment

It is as true for me that the practice of therapy has nourished my own religious
and personal values as much as my own religion, Judaism, has nourished and
influenced the therapy in which I participate. No longer for me do I favour
the monotheistic mode of participating in therapy, where one school of
therapy (psychoanalytic, behaviourist, systemic, among numerous others) is
paramount, perfect and absolute, with all other schools relegated to subordinate positions. Instead, as indicated in Section Two, I favour a pluralistic
view where, although all schools are valid, some are more effective and less
painful than others. Also very significant for me are the themes weaving
within the Jewish environment that is so much a part of my life: belonging
and permanence, the struggle for personal integration within a context of
community unity, a passion for human interaction, the search for social
equity, the strength of the family unit, and learning – oh, the excitement,
stimulation and joy of learning; learning from the old, learning within the
current experience! (Gunzburg 1991)

Martin Buber believed that learning was always gained through experiencing the world, through meeting in genuine dialogue within relationship
with others, never through analyzing and theorizing and thinking one's way
through the world in self-isolation. Buber's classic description of meeting is
that 'when two people meet in goodwill, the Shekhinah, the Divine Presence,
rests between them. The Hebrew word 'Shekhinah' is derived from the root
'to dwell', calling attention to the 'Divine Nearness'. In Jewish philosophy,
the Shekhinah denotes the Divine Presence which is manifest in the material
world; through learning, prayer and kindness to others, people can increase
their nearness to this Presence'. (Gunzburg and Stewart 1994).

Buber believed that through meeting, genuine dialogue and encountering
the Shekhinah, persons could increase their sense of wholeness and integra-

tion. For Buber, conversation was the context of human interaction. Words and ideas spoken were expressions of what people were experiencing. If we contemplate and examine the perspectives of a number of other explorers of mind and personality, contemplate the underlying themes that weave throughout their frameworks and explore how each attempted to explain how clients in therapy achieved wholeness and integration, we can conclude that what they were experiencing when they formulated their models of mind was not dissimilar to that which Buber experienced.

For Sigmund Freud, the context of human interaction was the *unconscious* (Strachey 1965). Freud developed the concept of conflict between a person's unconscious strivings and conscious awareness and how unconscious impulses influenced everyday activity. When people became overwhelmed by their unconscious struggles, Freud asserted that they were suffering from *neurotic* symptoms that preoccupied their time and created misery. Freud also described how, under stressful conditions, people would *regress* to infantile states from an earlier stage of personality development, and so be unable to cope in the adult world. These states of *neurosis* and *regression* very much parallel Buber's I–It position where a person thinks and behaves in concrete and self-focused ways and is unable to consider the needs of the other. Freud's methods of examination of his clients – psychoanalysis with a series of regular, frequent meetings of fifty-minute length, during which the client speaks freely and the therapist remains largely silent, and held over a period of some years – is much more formal than the encounters envisaged by Buber. The end result of psychoanalysis, however – in which the client recovers unconscious memories and, through this, gains 'insight' and is able to develop competence in his or her adult activities – does resemble Buber's I–Thou position in which clients feel included within society and confirmed in their personhood.

Ronald Laing (1965), like Buber, formulated his ideas within an *existential* context. Laing regarded Western technological society as one which *objectified* its members and disadvantaged their personal needs for the benefit of the collective needs of the group. To survive within such a society, Laing postulated, a person would have to develop a *false-self*, an outer personality that accommodated to the demands of society. The person's *true-self* (alive, inspirited, creative) would, over time, become overwhelmed by the *false-self* and eventually die. The *objectifying* society and *false-self* truly reflect Buber's I–It position, with persons within a group treating each other as things to be used, whilst the potential I–Thou position contained within the *true-self* remains imprisoned within them, unable to emerge. Laing accused Freud of contributing towards the objectification of people by using such labels as neurotic, narcissistic, obsessive and paranoid.

Carl Rogers (1975) and Abraham Maslow (1968) conceptualized their models within a *humanistic* context. Rogers termed the way that persons perceived themselves as their *self-structure*. This perception of themselves would grow over a period of time according to a person's experiences of the world. When a person's *self-structure* was *congruent* with his or her experience of the world, genuine expressions of feelings, attitudes and concerns for others were possible, as in the case of Buber's I–Thou position. When *self-structure* was *incongruent* with his or her experience of the world, psychological problems arose, for example anxiety, lack of confidence or disillusionment. Such psychological discomfort might induce persons to assume an I–It position, in which they might seek relief by exploiting others. Rogers felt that *congruency* between a person's *self-structure* and his or her experience of the world could be achieved within a genuine, warm, empathetic encounter with a *congruent* therapist, as in Buber's meeting within an I–Thou position, in which inclusion and confirmation occurred.

Maslow described people as advancing from an earlier developmental stage in the life process to a more mature adult phase in later life. During each of these stages, a person would have to achieve the needs of the stage before proceeding to the next one, that is they would have to achieve their physiological needs, then their needs for safety, for social contact, for self-esteem and, finally, for their needs for self-actualization. In Buber's terminology, when a person achieved competence at each stage, they might be described as confirming themselves, allowing them to strive for more complex tasks which also eventually become confirming in their achievement.

Erik Erikson (1968) viewed human growth within a *psycho-social* context. According to Erikson, people passed through several stages throughout their lifespan during which they learnt certain qualities that helped them to mature, that is, *basic trust* in infancy, *autonomy* as a toddler, *initiative* in kindergarten, *industry* in primary school, *identity* in adolescence, *intimacy* in young adulthood, *generativity* in middle age and *ego-integrity* in old age. Again, in Buber's approach, persons might be regarded as confirming their personhood through achieving the qualities of each stage.

Edward De Bono's (1970) interest is in how the human mind frames the knowledge that it receives. For De Bono, *Lateral* thinking (a person's ability to step outside a problem and consider it from a number of different angles) can be regarded as the context of *Vertical* or *Linear* thought (a person's ability to consider a number of bits of information and to narrow the data to one root cause). *Vertical* thinking can be considered to be De Bono's equivalent of Buber's I–It position, in which either/or logic narrows options and in which blaming of self or other can occur. *Lateral* thinking can be regarded as parallel to Buber's I–Thou position, in which there are increased options for relating differently: with compassion, understanding, co-operation and mutuality.

Gregory Bateson (Pentony 1981) elucidated five levels of learning. The lowest two levels were more concerned with people orienting themselves within their world spatially and sensorily. The middle level involved the symbolic nature of objects. The upper two levels, the most difficult to grasp, dealt with the metarules influencing the contexts within which people live. I have tabled Bateson's concept and have added two columns, one detailing the mode of learning at each of Bateson's levels and one illustrating how Buber's perspective approximates Bateson's hierarchical structure (Table 3.1)[1]

Table 3.1 The learning levels of Gregory Bateson and Buber's genuine dialogue

Bateson's Level of Learning	Characteristics of Bateson's levels of learning	Mode of learning at each of Bateson's levels	Buber's perspective
Learning Four	Context of Learning Three	Unattainable?	Approaching the Divine within an I–Thou position, spiritual confirmation
Learning Three	Context of Learning Two	Experiential	Meeting within an I–Thou position, confirmation
Learning Two	Context of Learning One: governs symbolic meanings of object	Analogic	Genuine dialogue, imagining the real, inclusion
Learning One	Context of Zero Learning: faster recognition of object	Digital	Meeting within an I–It position
Zero Learning	Initial learning details of object	Digital	Meeting within an I–It position

1   This Table is modified from Table 36.1 in Gunzburg (1991), p.228.

Consider an egg. Zero learning is the very first sighting of, and learning about, the egg: its size, shape, colour and consistency. Learning One is a faster recognition of the egg at second glance. This learning orients the observer to the object spatially and sensorily and is *digital* in nature: the object either is, or is not, an egg. For Buber, this can be considered the level at which participants initially commence their therapeutic conversation. By adopting the communally nominated roles of 'therapist' and 'client', participants can be regarded as meeting within an I–It position. It is not inherently disadvantageous to begin therapy within an I–It position, it only becomes so if these roles of therapist and client become rigid and unchanging throughout the duration of the conversation.

We therapists can be regarded as learning at Level One when we gather the tools of our trade, within our varied therapeutic schools. Psychoanalysts learn about projection, transference and free association (Freud 1960). Enmeshment, transactional patterns and sub-system boundaries make sense to family therapists (Minuchin 1974). Cognitive behaviourists talk of implosive techniques, treatment programmes and rational emotive therapy 'musterbation' (Ellis 1987). Our patients can also be considered as spending much of their time during therapy learning at these levels: identifying, recognizing and defining the emotions, thoughts, feelings and behaviours that trouble them.

Learning Two consists of the context which determines the symbolic meaning of the object. In Judaism, the Passover egg is a marker for an eternal nation, given to life from bondage through God's Laws (Ben Asher 1979). To Christians, it is an Easter egg of resurrection and salvation through Christ (Williams 1979). The pagan ovum is a salutation to the Teutonic goddess Oestre, fertile and abundant (May 1970). So, rather than the either/or (egg/not egg) perspective of Learning One, at Learning Two level we have a both/and (egg as object/egg as symbol within a context) framework; one egg, the same shape, size and texture, and three contexts, rich and varied. Within Buber's perspective, Bateson's Learning Two can be considered the level where therapists enter a genuine dialogue which includes both themselves and their clients, imagining the real of their clients' situation and inviting clients to consider that there is more than one context within which to view their struggles.

Our schools of therapy are also rich and varied yet, like the Jewish, Christian and Pagan peoples throughout history, we battle to determine which context is the Absolute and Right One. In Buber's terminology, those therapists who battle for ideological supremacy against their colleagues, can be considered as acting within an I–It position: they, the infallible therapists, struggle to impose their inflexible therapeutic framework onto those of their colleagues and clients. Those colleagues and clients can thus be regarded as being objectified by the therapists, each being considered an 'It', and having to fit into the framework of the 'all-knowing experts'. Though our schools do differ in mythology, ritual and text, we can be regarded as achieving a like function at the level of Learning Two. At Bateson's Learning Level Two, we can be considered as creating a nourishing environment within which our patients can reflect, grow and heal. Our patients present within their own contexts (often viewing themselves and others within an I–It position, with decreased options for change) and we can contact them within our contexts (hopefully holistic in character, viewing our clients within an I–Thou position and with expanded options for change).

Bateson's Learning Three is the context of Learning Two. It can be regarded as the level of the hypnotic trance (Edelstein 1981), the therapeutic anecdote (Haley 1973) and the family dance (Whitaker and Napier 1978) where intrapsychic and interactional perspectives meet. It is the level of I–Thou meeting, where contraries reconcile, analytic and intuitive modes of thinking co-operate (Ornstein 1975) and where syntheses occur – as in my writing this essay: serious contemplation combined with a playful and creative imagination. It is the level of learning where we often have most fun, and where magic happens! It is also where we make the paradoxical leap to a new dimension and experience: 'Ah-Ha! We therapists are all talking about exactly the same thing!'

Learning Three also contains the metarules regulating the contexts within Learning Two. I believe that among those metarules is how we choose the contexts within which we function best. We can be considered to do this from an experiential learning of what regulates our patients within their contexts and what regulates us within our contexts. First, we can be regarded as being influenced by intrapsychic needs. Returning to our egg as symbol, people may have a desire for belonging, permanence and continuity within an ethnocentric group (Judaism), hunger for personal immortality through Jesus (Christianity) or yearn to be made whole through contact with pantheistic Nature (Paganism). Second, I believe that Bateson's Learning Three represents the level at which we develop an ethical awareness of the consequences of change upon our relationships. For instance, it would be too disruptive on my current family life for me to trade the egg of the Chosen People for one promising a Christian Paradise regained. There would be too many connections severed within my social network to exchange my present Jewish values for a pagan stance. In similar fashion, I believe that it is essential for us therapists to develop an ethical awareness about which outcomes are most likely to benefit each particular client (so that we do not view our clients continually within an I–It position) and as to which therapeutic contexts will produce the most useful outcomes. It is not enough for therapists to collect a bag of tricks of spectrum of clever techniques! I believe that we must learn to work effectively within a variety of therapeutic frameworks. So, for me, Bateson's Learning Level Three can be considered an understanding and choosing of contexts. It is the level of ethical action, at which we learn to match our personal desires with the needs of our environment. It is an accommodating to the many systems of 'being' without becoming accommodated by them. It involves a partial dissolution of self and ego. It is an experiential event which includes tolerance, trust, respect and compassion for individuals within specific and differing systems, and which embraces a love of human interaction across boundaries. It is living within an ecology, contacting intimate others from other domains of being.

In Buber's view, Learning Three concerns a shift in position from I–It to I–Thou. The roles of therapist and client can be regarded as dissipating. Clients and therapists can confirm each other as existential equals, travelling as participants within the same journey. Generally, it is at this point where clients, having experienced enough of meeting their therapists within an I–Thou position and feeling confident that they can achieve an I–Thou position within their intimate network, leave therapy.

Finally, to Learning Level Four. Bateson claims that we never achieve it (for who can see the Face of God and live?) and that perhaps only computers of the future will have the capacity to comprehend the context (Learning Four) of the context (Learning Three) regulating contexts (Learning Two).

Yet if we cannot comprehend Learning Four, perhaps we can apprehend it. For me, Learning Four is the wholeness and integration that we endeavour to achieve within our lifespan, both personally and communally.

There are many metaphors describing this idea: a Unity of experience, the One, God, the Absolute Good of Plato, the Hindu atman becoming Brahma, the Christ in us all, the Nothingness of Buddha (Watts 1975), the Jewish Shekinah – a Divine Presence felt when two persons meet in goodwill (Gunzburg and Stewart 1994) – the empathic encounter of Carl Rogers (Rogers 1975), Martin Buber's genuine dialogue (Friedman 1960), Ronald Laing's communion of true selves (Laing 1965) – a union of persons choosing their contexts yet transcending those contexts by their very act of choosing – Yin interlocking with Yang (Wilhelm 1967), the 'egoless state' and Unconscious made known, with contraries reconciled (Jacobi 1973). To grasp these metaphors as a collective expression of a common universal experience can be regarded as abandoning that religious love in which people kill one another and approaching Bateson's Learning Level Four. Buber might say that this is the level where we come close to God, where the material world is nullified (through meditation, prayer, singing in unison, trance states) and we experience the Divine, confirming ourselves as spiritual beings. A reality in therapy today is that we therapists do share that religious zeal with which persons kill one another! Psychodynamic practitioners and systems thinkers tussle against one another – as do psychoanalysts against brief (future-focused) therapists, social constructivists against post-modernists and psychiatrists against non-medically trained therapists. Our contexts, our various therapeutic schools, do seem to be battling for ideological supremacy. We appear to be abandoning our quest for wholeness. In the Hebrew language there is a word that I believe approaches Learning Four: 'Shleymoos', meaning wholeness, perfection and being a cousin to 'Shalom', peace.

So, let us cease our wars promoting the welfare of the false gods Theoretical Bias, Slick Technique and Absolute Truth. Let us honour our therapeutic frameworks, just as we talk about respecting our clients' worlds of being. Our therapeutic perspectives can be regarded as different ways of structuring and processing our experience. How can we colleagues learn about each other's contexts with humour, creativity and cross-fertilization of each other's views at Learning Level Three? How can we participate together within an I–Thou structure that is nourishing to clients, therapists and colleagues alike and that sets us in process towards the uniting and universal intimacy of Learning Four? For those persons who denied that the 'oneness', alluded to in Learning Level Four, approximated the ground of our being, Gregory Bateson liked to quote the Lord answering Job out of the whirlwind:

> Who is this that darkeneth counsel by words without knowledge...
> Where was thou when I laid the foundations of the earth?
>
> Declare if thou hast understanding... (Job 38, 2–4)

The quality of the therapeutic conversation

The *Family Counselling Casebook* (Gunzburg 1991) took up Bateson's ideas on Levels of Learning and incorporated them into a schema that considered the quality of the therapeutic conversation. A suggestion was made that our clients entered therapy to learn about themselves at different levels. They can be regarded as wishing to:

- Define exactly what their problems are (the descriptive level of learning; Bateson's Learning Level One)

- Become more familiar with the context in which their problems arose or were currently occurring (the contextual level of learning; Bateson's Learning Level Two)

- Achieve a resolution of their problems and expand their world-view, utilizing their own choices and resources (the experiential level of learning; Bateson's Learning level Three).

At the experiential level of learning, a nourishing environment was considered to be created – involving warmth, empathy, clear yet permeable boundaries, a definite sense of self and a genuine liking for people. In such an atmosphere, clients were regarded as exploring, growing, changing and healing. Clients could learn to cease being overly preoccupied with their own problems and interact within a wider social community. Learning at this level was considered to be mutual, although therapists were held to be responsible for all changes made as being in their clients' best interest, that is maintaining clients' safety, dignity, independence, autonomy, enabling them to contest the various abuses which they might be facing in their lives and increasing their flexibility of choices. Therapists would have to be open to their own learning processes during the therapeutic encounter. Some of the ways that therapists could best foster experiential learning were thought to be: offering insight (Freud 1960), enabling self-actualization (Maslow 1968) and expression of the 'true self' (Laing 1965), encouraging congruency and accurate expression of feelings (Rogers 1975), engaging in an intimate dialogue where values could be defined and dilemmas discussed (Friedman 1960) and the use of reframing (Watzlawick, Weakland and Fisch 1974). Humour and a playful imagination, as well as serious contemplation and the knowledge of a number of therapeutic models, were considered essential.

Unresolved Grief (Gunzburg 1993) further developed the concept that the quality of the therapeutic conversation can be enhanced if these three basic levels of learning are incorporated within it:

1. Defining the problem: There is, initially, a descriptive level of discussion during which therapists and their clients together explore and define the emotions, thoughts and behaviours with which the latter are struggling (Therapists who find themselves battling with the same feelings in their personal lives as their clients may need to focus on their own dilemmas within their own supervision, peer interchange or therapy so that their own personal agenda doesn't impinge on that of their clients). Questions during the descriptive discussion are usually open-ended and non-specific

and geared to elicit information as to how clients are experiencing their problems: What is happening in your life at the moment? What has brought you along to therapy? How can I be of help to you? This descriptive level of discussion can be regarded as occurring at Bateson's Learning Level One. Clients often describe their feelings, behaviours and thoughts as things that are happening to them, that they are experiencing, in either/or terms; either this or that is happening to them. This can also be considered a conversation within Buber's I–It position. Often, at this stage of therapy, clients will be filled with blame – either of themselves, or others. They appear to regard themselves as an 'It', helpless to resolve their dilemmas, or they consider their intimates as 'It', incapable of change. As discussed earlier, it is important for therapists not to slot clients into one particular therapeutic school, to be used on all clients who attend, for fear of increasing the clients' sense of being an 'It' but rather to listen carefully to clients, tuning in to their nuances and unique qualities. In so doing, therapists and clients can *meet* and therapists can more readily invite clients into a *genuine dialogue*.

2. Exploring the context: There is next a contextual level of discussion within which therapists and their clients endeavour to understand the ground against which the troublesome emotions,thoughts and behaviours evolved and the current situation that maintains their existence. Questions at this level are usually more specific in seeking the details surrounding the problem: When was the first time that you noticed this problem? When did you learn to respond like this? Who else is involved in this? The contextual level of discussion can be regarded as occurring at Bateson's Learning Level Two, at which the contexts of both therapists and clients need to be acknowledged and addressed. For Buber, this can be considered the stage of therapeutic conversation where therapists, in '*imagining the real* aspects of their clients' world, can encourage *inclusion* of both themselves and their clients within the conversation.

3. Options for the future: Finally, there is an experiential level of discussion during which clients seek a resolution of their struggles whilst experiencing trust, safety, autonomy, adequate boundaries, appropriate closeness-distance between therapists and clients, co-operation, development of mutuality and reflection. During this

phase, clients are encouraged to search for those resources that are available to them and the ethical options that exist to promote future change, growth and healing: Have you ever handled this situation in a different manner? Do you know of anyone who has tackled the problem differently? Would you speak about it with him/her? What are your strengths, talents, spiritual resources? Buber's ideas correspond very readily with those of Bateson within the this schema.

The experiential level of discussion can be regarded as occurring at Bateson's Learning Level Three and Buber's I–Thou position; where *contraries* are *reconciled* and both therapists and clients are *confirmed* in their wholeness of being. From this position, therapists and clients can apprehend Learning Level Four: Bateson's 'oneness' that is the ground of human experience and which for Buber represented the highest possible I–Thou position: an authentic intimacy with God – a circumstance which Buber termed *Grace* (Buber 1958).

Structuring tales of empowerment

I often share stories with clients to illustrate a specific aspect of the therapeutic conversation and/or to highlight he many complex themes that can be found weaving within human interaction. However, for tales to be empowering, it can be useful to follow a certain structure:

1. Commence with a descriptive section: what is troubling clients? How do they define their struggle? Use the same terminology that clients use. This is similar to the early part of the therapeutic conversation, during which therapists follow the pace of their clients, using similar energy, body postures, voice tones and language as their clients to encourage connectedness. In so doing, story-tellers can convey to their listeners the atmosphere in which therapists and clients commenced to meet.

2. Continue with a section which details how contexts are explored. The story-teller can illustrate how the focus of conversation changes away from clients blaming themselves or others (viewing themselves and others within an I–It position) towards viewing the problem within a wider context which includes therapists, clients and their intimates. In this part of the story, therapists can detail how they imagined the real, what their reflections were about what clients were saying and how therapists visualized another

facet of the clients' lives which might be highlighted usefully within the therapeutic conversation.

3. Conclude with a section which describes signs of change over the period of therapy. Ideally, this should include details of the outcome some months later but this is not always possible. Sometimes clients improve very rapidly and it is worthwhile to tell a story about how clients changed during that particular therapeutic conversation but, some time later, therapists may find that the clients have relapsed or are struggling with a new problem. Therapy can be regarded as helping clients to move from one set of problems to another in which the struggles are easier.

Stories can be told:

- To encourage meeting: In Case 2Z (p.97), Gary and the therapist met through the therapist reaching out and putting a hand of comfort on the disconsolate Gary's shoulder.

- To clarify an issue: In Case 1F (p.20), Marnie communicated her reaction to her parent's divorce clearly through her drawing of the family.

- To include clients within the human drama: In Case 2S (p.82), Joyce blames herself as 'stupid and weak' for remaining in her abusive relationship with Don and alienating her family. She is invited to reflect on her distress within a wider social context: the patriarchal themes that have influenced men in their oppression of women, and which women can contest in regaining their own empowerment. These themes can be regarded as widespread throughout the whole western world (Walters *et al.* 1988).

- To achieve balance whenever clients are skewed towards one contrary position: In Case 1D (p.12), Thelma, a structured mathematical thinker, is invited to use the intuitive side of her psyche to resolve her struggles.

Stories can be empowering by:

- Inviting listeners to track the changes within the telling and to compare them to their own situation: In Case 2J (p.59), many aspects of the therapeutic conversation is clearly presented in this essay and clients can be invited to consider, and feel free in commenting upon, any changes made.

○ Including both listeners and tellers within the human drama: in Cases 2O, 2P and 2Q (pp.72–5), the struggles of clients and therapist are presented in parallel. Such stories include therapists and clients within the whole human fabric and it can be enormously liberating for clients to realise that their therapists are also human!

○ Contesting injustices: In Case 2T (p.59), the therapist brings into focus Myra's harsh treatment of herself in continuing to live up to the unrealistically high expectations of her family of origin. It can be empowering for clients to be invited to rewrite an unjust script that has been composed for them by others in their past when they were growing up, and even before they were born.

○ Clarifying a certain point: In Case 2F (p.42), Brko is invited to consider whether grief remaining from his father's past abuse underlies his feelings of rage, rather than some psychiatric disorder. Clarifying issues can free clients to make more effective decisions about their lives.

○ Giving hope that change can occur: In Case 2J (p.59), Lesley is invited to consider that she is not 'mad', but that her 'Unconscious' is retrieving information from her past. Discovering hidden resources can liberate clients from their traps and can renew their confidence for the future.

○ Getting a different angle on an issue: In Case 1A (p.7), Cal and Sylvie's arguments are reframed as trying to negotiate and they are asked to define how they knew they 'cared' about each other. After this, Cal and Sylvie appeared to acknowledge that they were both different from, yet interested in, each other. In recognizing both their differences and their similarities, clients can be feel free to negotiate that their needs to be met.

Although all the case studies in this book have been included with the specific aim of therapists sharing them with their clients to facilitate the therapeutic conversation, in Section Three the stories have been composed particularly to 'constitute help in themselves'. I shall continue to present, however, a brief discussion section at the end of each case study inviting readers to reflect on the structure underlying each story and on Buber's ideas that weave throughout the text: meeting, genuine dialogue, I–It and I–Thou positions, imagining the real, inclusion, reconciling contraries and confirmation.

Case 3A: Taking charge[2]

April, 1993: Hannah, 48 years, was grieving the loss of her job of twenty-four years as administrative clerk three weeks previously. Usually a conscientious and effective worker, Hannah had gradually lost energy, become depressed and unable to concentrate or co-operate with her colleagues for the past several months. Her decreased work performance had led to early retirement on sickness benefits.

Hannah's childhood had been a horrible one. Her mother, Ruby, now 72, had been a strict disciplinarian who had locked the youthful Hannah in a wardrobe overnight as a punishment for a perceived misdemeanour. The father, James, who had died in 1992, had often gone outside and had tossed large pebbles onto the corrugated roof of their house. As the stones had rumbled down the metal slope, Ruby would tell Hannah that the sound was that of 'the Devil coming to punish naughty children'. James had sexually abused Hannah when she was 11. When Hannah was 22, her elder brother Peter was brain-damaged in a motor vehicle accident. Not only was Hannah grieving the loss of her job, and blaming herself as 'a weak person who was letting the community down', she did not seem able to prevent the neighbours from exploiting her. Dave, 55, an aged pensioner, frequently borrowed Hannah's utensils – a television, a vacuum cleaner – and failed to return them. Irina, 58, a widow, was badgering Hannah to let her move in permanently. Irina had even marked Hannah's bedroom as her own, encouraging Hannah to sleep on the couch in the lounge.

Our conversation focused on how Hannah had been devalued and discounted in her family of origin. I was admiring that despite James and Ruby's cruel abuse and lack of protection during her childhood, Hannah had determined to participate in the work-force for many decades. Perhaps her 'depression' was a message from her psyche, indicating that Hannah now needed to take some 'time out', to concentrate on healing herself and develop her own emotional security? We discussed ways of negotiating with Dave; Hannah decided that he could keep the vacuum cleaner but return the television set. Dave acceded to Hannah's wishes. Hannah said that she had told Irina she was contented with her own company and wanted to continue living alone. Irina had stopped harassing Hannah. After eighteen months of weekly therapy, Hannah is no longer depressed, and is seeking further employment.

---

2   This case was originally presented in the 'General Practitioner', *Adis International 2*, 3, February–March 1994, 19.

Discussion

The 'developmental map' can be regarded as the context of the therapeutic conversation: exploring how Hannah had experienced a lengthy history of childhood abuse and deprivation. Nonetheless, despite the violations of her caretakers (who could be considered to have viewed Hannah within an I–It position, using her as a receptacle for their negative feelings), Hannah had managed to hold employment for many years and the economic recession, rather than any personal weakness, could be regarded as having resulted in the loss of her job. Therapy aimed to:

1. Promote an environment in which Hannah could feel safe and heard and be able to tell her story (this can be regarded as the phase of therapeutic conversation during which meeting and the commencement of genuine dialogue took place. Hannah used words which enabled the therapist to imagine the real of her world: lost energy, depressed, unable to concentrate or co-operate, decreased work performance, a weak person, a failure, letting the community down).

2. Affirm her strength in being able to survive (this can be considered a confirmation of Hannah as a resourceful person).

3. Invite Hannah to shift her perception away from her being 'too weak to work' to requiring 'some time to heal self'(this can be regarded as inclusion. Hannah was invited to cease viewing herself within an I–It position, calling herself 'weak' and 'a failure', and to join the human race within an I–Thou position: we all need, I believe, some time to contemplate our lot and ease our stresses).

4. Develop some assertiveness skills so that Hannah can lay down some boundaries round her emotional territory and have her own needs met (during this phase of therapy, Hannah can be seen as confirming herself).

5. Reconciling of the contraries: weakness/strength, and failure/success, can also be considered to have occurred here. Hannah blames herself as 'weak, and a failure', in not being able to work but the therapist describes her as a 'strong survivor of abuse' and 'successfully knowing when she needs to rest herself and heal'. The therapist's views can be regarded as countering Hannah's disesteeming self-criticism and inviting her to enter another perspective in which she can feel empowered and liberated.

When I read this story out to Hannah. she responded: 'It doesn't sound so frightening when you read it like that'.

Case 3B: Fourth past the post[3]

November, 1993: The Melbourne Cup (Australia's premier horse race) had just been run and won by Vintage Crop. Louise, 44 years, who had gained a diploma in primary education but was currently unemployed due to a work injury, recounted yet another disappointment with her interstate lover, Tim, 45, a university professor in Social Sciences. Tim had promised to come for the weekend but was now telling Louise that pressures from work, his wife, Jenny, 45, and their two children, Bart, 19, and Lisa, 17, were forcing him to cancel it. Such reversals had occurred many times in the past. Moreover, Tim seemed to be using Louise as an 'easy lay' when visiting Melbourne on business, rarely telephoning her or sending her messages of affection for her birthday, Christmas, etc.

During the first months of weekly therapy, it became apparent that Louise had come from a conservative, rural, formally religious family in which there had been no fun. Life was all hard work on the farm. Louise's father had been an authoritarian, directive, abusive patriarch and she and her mother appeared to have entered the roles of 'caring for and protecting one other' against the father's cruel taunts. Louise had also faced much humiliation at primary school during which she had developed a poor self-image. I asked Louise if she would write a letter contesting her father's abuse. Louise wrote:

> This is a letter to tell you how much I detest/loathe/hate the way you treated Mum and all of us (your children) especially Tony and myself. Mum worked day and night for you and us with not ONCE a thank you, any verbal recognition, no money or gifts in 40 years. She had NOTHING, but to be treated like a dog (which was treated badly too) or a slave.
>
> Tony and I both were treated like child slaves. We were only in Grade 3 and 4 and you had us helping you milk the cows. You could have done it by yourself. We were only children. Then when Mum went to the cow-shed on my behalf, I was expected to look after the twins (and later Charles), clean up after afternoon tea, cook tea (chops and vegetables), and bath twins (once a week in used water, no shower). In the mornings, besides myself, I had to make sure the table was set chiefly for you. Everything had to be at your beck and call or you would be moaning and criticizing and yelling. I had to prepare 4

---

3   This case was originnally presented in the 'General Practitioner', *Adis International 2*, 3, February–March, 1994, 19.

lunches (later 6) and have/get my own breakfast. Noone could be having a bath (or you would interrupt) or be using the hand-basin (or you would push/knock/yell at them) the first minute you returned from milking. Noone was allowed to speak while the news was on – you might miss a syllable. If it was raining, you would never drive us to the bus stop or let Mum. We would just have to run and get wet. I remember I was the one who had to collect the local paper Monday/Wednesday/Friday and whoa betide if I forgot sometimes (very rarely). You would moan and groan and criticize and if you could, pull my ear and/or swipe at my head (but on those occasions, I never left Mum's side because she was often my shelter).

You – had no respect, swore often, physically hit the cows and dog, moaned and groaned and criticized when Mum bought us new shoes, pencils, etc. for school, gave us no books, gave us toys only at Xmas, gave us no birthday parties or presents, made Mum cut our hair, moaned and groaned and criticized whenever (every month, I think) I had to visit the eye doctor to have an infection treated. You never took me, very rarely got us new clothes, and if we did, you moaned and groaned and criticized. We always had second-hand beds/dressing tables/furniture and never enough blankets and overcoats to keep us warm. You never ever said a pleasant word to any of us children, but you put on a good show if anyone came to visit. The minute you got out of bed (before you even said your prayers) you woke me, then Tony (I don't ever remember you wakening Mary). When you killed a sheep, after cutting it into appropriate sections, I (Mum would be milking) would have to clean up your bloody mess and put the meat in the refrigerator. You fronted up to Mass on Sunday but never said or did a Christian thing all week.

Louise and I discussed whether her affair with Tim had initially been an exploration in 'breaking the rules', 'having fun' and 'developing a sense of self'. Over the next several months, I encouraged Louise to explore relationships within Melbourne that gave her a greater permanence and continuity of enjoyment. Tim continued to see her every four to six weeks but his visits were unpredictable and fraught with insecurity and anxiety for Louise. Louise them met Derek, 48, an industrial engineer, whose wife had died six years previously. Derek was nervous about committing himself to a new relationship but Louise said that they were obviously attracted to one another and she enjoyed the feelings of affection and companionship with Derek that she had only experienced in her intimacy with Tim. 'Look at the difference', I commented. 'If your friendship with Tim was the Melbourne Cup, you would not get a place. Past the post would be: Tim – first; Tim's work –

second; Tim's family – third; Tim's lover, Louise – fourth! At least with Derek you have a chance of influencing the direction of your relationship. With Tim you have been lagging in the race for years'.

Three months later, Louise says that she is preparing to 'give Tim the flick' and that she and Derek are warming to each other.

Discussion

Louise told of her sense of disempowerment in her relationship with Tim. The 'developmental map' can be regarded as the therapeutic context within which Louise was encouraged to examine the abusive model of masculinity that her father had presented to her in her youth. The father appeared to have viewed Louise within an I–It position, regarding Louise as being there to tend to his beck and call. Now Tim seemed to be repeating this disrespectful model. In the letter which contested her father's violations, Louise used words that made it easy for the therapist to imagine the real of her world: detest, loathe, hate, child slaves, push, knock, yell, moan, groan, criticize. Louise's affair with Tim was framed as an effort to find some of the fun and 'naughtiness' that she missed out on in her youth. This can be regarded as a reconciliation of the contraries: autonomy/shame and initiative/guilt. Louise appeared to have been raised in an environment where any ordinary effort to assert her independence would have been treated as a disgraceful event. Reframing the affair as an attempt to establish her freedom and an effort to discard the limiting patterns of relating which she had learnt in her family of origin can be regarded as an invitation to Louise to stop blaming herself and choose less painful ways to achieve her independence. Louise's writing the letter, and the therapist inviting Louise to consider her affair as a quest for happiness, can also be considered acts of inclusion; I believe that all survivors of abuse should be offered the opportunity to contest the violence that they have experienced and that we can all be considered explorers in our lives, searching for qualities that will enrich our lives. A more recent and accessible friendship with Derek was explored, confirming Louise's abilities to enter more successful intimate relationships.

When I shared this story with Louise, she responded:' But why am I the only member of the family to moan and groan and criticize about Dad's behaviour?' I invited Louise to consider that perhaps her moaning and groaning and criticizing expressed her desire for positive change in the family whereas her father's moaning and groaning and criticizing represented his dumping of his bad feelings onto her.

Case 3C: Possessed[4,5]

March, 1989: Melanie, 21 years, a student at one of Melbourne's colleges of the arts, was telling me of her interchangeable moods. At times she would experience weeks of depression, 'black holes with no bottom to them', during which she would lose all her energy and her ability to work. Melanie's entrance to therapy was during one such episode when she had absented herself from drama classes for two weeks. On other occasions, Melanie would experience 'buzzing' in her head, 'lots of noises, at all different pitches and levels', associated with frantic activity to complete her chores. At these times, Melanie would rage throughout the night with friends, smoke marijuana, get drunk and generally spend a life of carefree abandon. Melanie's mother was diagnosed some years before as a manic depressive. She was prescribed lithium and had been stable on this medication for three years. Melanie wondered if she might be heading down the same track.

As twice-weekly therapy progressed, our conversation turned to the rather rigorous training that Melanie had experienced during her teenage years in a convent. 'I was always having a go at the nuns', Melanie said, 'I couldn't hack the idea of the immaculate conception and the infallibility of the Pope. No bloody man was going to tell me how to run my sex life! They all thought that I was a pretty bad case but then the priest thought that I had been possessed by the devil. I would always vomit when I swallowed the host during Mass. It went on for a couple of years. Mum and the doctors thought that I was developing anorexia but the priest was certain that it was Satan's work. I think that, in desperation, he had worked out some sort of exorcism. But, right from the start, I knew what was wrong with me. They had taught us that the host became part of Jesus' body at the moment of eating it and I could not come at the idea of cannibalism. The thought of digesting human flesh really made me feel sick! But I wasn't going to tell them. It all stopped when I was sixteen and decided to give up the Church for good. I have never been to Mass since – and have never vomited again when eating anything.'

Discussion

This is an excellent example of how offering a client space to speak can encourage genuine dialogue and meeting. Melanie can be regarded as telling her story within the context of the 'developmental map': recounting how she made sense of what was happening to her during her adolescence. It was

4   Another story about Melanie was told in Gunzburg 1991, pp.251–2.
5   This case was originally presented in the 'General Practitioner', *Adis International 2*, 9, May 1994, 9–10.

not difficult for me to imagine the real of Melanie's world considering the words she used: black holes with no bottom in them, depression, loss of energy and ability to work, buzzing and lots of noises inside the head. If I had not listened to Melanie's whole account, I might easily have labelled her, within an I–It position, as psychotic! The priest had thought that Melanie was infested by evil spirits but Melanie appeared to know herself better. Rather than being possessed, she defined herself as resisting the rigid, fundamentalist aspects of her faith. This can be considered as a reconciling of contraries: autonomy/shame and identity/identity diffusion. The priest can be regarded as wanting to designate Melanie, within an I–It position, as 'possessed, shameful, bad', whereas Melanie can be considered as acknowledging herself, within an I–Thou position, as a maturing adult well able to reject those tenets of her religion which she held unpalatable. Melanie's nausea can be regarded as an act of confirmation of her identity during her adolescence; her vomiting disappeared when she changed her beliefs.

Case 3D: Humiliation[6]

September, 1993: Michael, 41 years, a business executive, was distraught that he was sexually impotent with his lover of three months, Lim, 38, an industrial engineer. Michael had been married for thirteen years to Geraldine, 42, also an executive, and they had one son, Peter, 11. Michael described his marriage as having lost its 'special quality' ever since their son's birth. He had met and felt immediately attracted to Lim. This was not the first time that Michael had been erotically aroused by his own gender but it was the first time that he had acted on such feelings. It had proved to be a warm, accepting, companionate relationship quite unlike anything he had ever experienced with Geraldine, so Michael was distressed that he could not extend these feelings into the physical arena. Michael said that Geraldine had no idea that he had become involved in an extramarital affair. I suggested to Michael that perhaps his problem was an ethical one rather than a biological or psychological one. Was there any 'unfinished business' between himself and Geraldine, and how could he cement his friendship with Lim before he completed such business? I asked Michael if he would invite his wife to our next meeting.

When Michael and Geraldine attended together a week later, Michael re-stated his unhappiness with the situation. He felt that the onus was on him to change but also that changes would be required of his wife. Geraldine responded that she did think that 'it was Michael's problem' and that,

---

6   This case was originally presented in the 'General Practitioner', *Adis International 2, 9*, May 1994, 9–10.

basically, she was contented in her lot. She and Michael did share a number of activities together: science fiction films, visiting restaurants with friends, as well as many outings on her own. It did not appear to bother Geraldine that they had not participated in lovemaking for two years. Geraldine said that she felt no need to attend another joint session and that Michael should 'sort himself out'. If he was happier, she would be happier.

At our next meeting, with Michael attending on his own, he spoke of his sense of loneliness and isolation within the family. He had become particularly irritated at Peter, who was used to spending most Sunday mornings reading in bed with Geraldine whilst Michael was up and about working around the house. The previous Sunday, when Michael had decided to rest in bed until noon, Peter had come into their bedroom and said to his mother: 'Is that man going to stay in our bed this morning?'. I expressed my concern that Geraldine and Peter were developing a depth of relationship that is usually found within the emotional territory of intimate couples. My apprehension was that if such a relationship persisted, Peter would have a difficult time achieving his independence as a young adult when the time came. Perhaps this circumstance was one of the factors influencing Michael to seek contact outside the marriage? Had he felt excluded from closeness within his marriage and endeavoured to find it with Lim? I wondered if there would be any advantage gained in seeing Michael and Peter together?

Michael and I continued to meet weekly, during which time he discussed his experiences within his family of origin. Michael's father appeared to have been a directive parent, always telling Michael what to do. I queried whether the father had genuinely cared for his son or had he been intrusive and dominating, raising Michael to be a little clone of himself? Both father and mother appeared to have been continually criticizing and discounting of each other without resolving their differences. Did Michael learn early that some families have to put up with unresolved situations that grind round and round forever? Was that why he was tolerating the situation with Geraldine and Peter, believing that this was the best family life he could get? At our eighth session, Michael and Peter both attended. Peter was a beautifully groomed, quiet, sad little lad who said that he did not believe that his father cared much about him. Michael burst into tears at this point and told Peter that this was the way that he felt about his own father, and said that he had worked so hard to spare Peter the same experience but nothing seemed to have worked. There was another point also: Michael described how he used to yell at Peter incessantly when the boy was younger – 'Why are you taking so long in the bath? Aren't you dressed yet? My God, you're a slow eater!' This is exactly the way Michael's father had humiliated him and it had only just occurred to Michael, with full impact, how humiliated Peter must have felt when Michael had behaved in this manner. I asked Michael if he would express his regrets to Peter now that he had acted in such a demeaning fashion towards his son. Michael did so without hesitation. We discussed how humiliation leads to feelings of sadness, low self-esteem, poor self-image, loss of confidence. I asked Michael if he would write a Certificate of Non-Humiliation, declaring his intent never to treat Peter, or anyone else, in this way in the future. Michael agreed to do so. Peter sat up several inches straighter in his chair and I saw him smile for the first time.

Michael and I continued to meet after this session, during which we discussed ways of being assertive without being aggressive. I gave him Erich Fromm's *The Art of Loving* (1957) to peruse. I also shared with Michael one of my favourite passages quoted from the writings of Milton D. Erickson:

> When I describe a good marriage to my patients, I point out to them that there are essentially four kinds of love. The infantile type of love, 'I love me'. The next stage, 'I love the me in you, I love you because you are my brother, my mother, my father, my sister, my dog. The me in you'. Then the adolescent type of love. 'I love you because your dancing pleases me, and because your beauty pleases me, and because your brains please me'. And the adult stage of love wherein, 'I want to love you and cherish you because I want to see you happy because I can find my happiness in your happiness. The happier you are, the happier I'll be. I find my happiness in yours. I'll find my delight in your pleasure and intellectual pursuits. I'll find a delight in your enjoyment of dancing'. So, the mature love is the capacity to find enjoyment in the enjoyment of the other person's enjoyment. It works both ways. (Haley 1985, p.121)

Michael said that, for the first time in his life, he felt free to make space for himself and tend to his own needs.

Six months later, Michael and Geraldine were negotiating their separation. Michael, whose impotence had disappeared some weeks after he had commenced therapy, had also negotiated an ending to the sexual relationship with Lim, saying that he needed some time on his own, away from all intimate relationships, to find himself. They remain friends. As it happened, Lim had also been interested in pursuing a partnership with a female colleague for some time and had not known how to tell Michael for fear of hurting him. Michael said that although Peter still shared his mother's bed on Sundays, he had become much more open to time spent with his father. I suggested that after Michael and Geraldine separated, Geraldine and Peter might well 'rebalance' their relationship and find intimate support within their respective peer groups. After a further three months, Michael told me that he and Geraldine had agreed to a property settlement amicably and that Peter was 'out of the bedroom'. Michael said that he had recently gained his motorcycle driver's licence, something which he had always contemplated but had never felt confident enough to achieve.

Michael's Certificate of Non-Humiliation:

I, Michael Smith, promise -

1) not to inflict hurt or pain on anyone else.

2) not to laugh at someone else's hurt or pain.

3) not to use humiliation to encourage or change someone else's behaviour.

4) to check out if it is okay to enjoy a 'silly' incident. It may not always be appropriate to enjoy a 'silly' incident. Others may not understand and it could lead them to cry.

5) to check out the context of enjoying a 'silly' incident. It might be okay within the family or with close friends, but not in broader company. Some 'silly' incidents may always be better ignored. Sometimes laughter just means relief that everything is okay. Laughing is sometimes a way to reduce the hurt or pain. I will always let others know that I am laughing WITH them and not AT them.

Discussion

The 'developmental, systemic and structural maps' can be regarded as the therapeutic contexts used to explore how Michael first experienced humiliation, how his relationships with Lim, Geraldine and Peter are impinging on one another, and what structure the family might adopt in the future so there is less hurt for them all? Michael used words that enabled the therapist to imagine the real of his world: distraught, unhappy, isolated, loneliness, having lost the 'specialness' within his marriage, impotence. Michael seemed to consider the decreased sexual competence with his lover as his main problem but I invited him to contemplate that his struggle was whether he could invest in a new relationship without resolving his current one. This invitation can be regarded as exploring a reconciliation of the contrary: intimacy/ isolation. Michael might have to resolve his sense of detachment within his relationships with Geraldine and Peter before achieving a stable intimacy with Lim or, indeed, anyone else. Michael revealed areas of his past experience: that families never resolve their conflicts and that life is filled with humiliation. During a conversation with Peter, Michael acknowledged his past humiliation of his son and pledged a course towards future reconciliation with him. Those who humiliated Michael can be regarded as having viewed him within an I–It position, just as Michael can be considered to have viewed Peter within an I–It position when he had tormented his son. By writing his Certificate of Non-Humiliation, Michael can be considered as moving into an I–Thou position with Peter. Michael said that he also felt more liberated to negotiate new directions with both his wife and lover, perhaps having moved into an I–Thou position with them, since this event. The session with Peter and Michael particularly can be regarded as an act of meeting, genuine dialogue and inclusion: both participants conversing to understand each other's view, recognizing past injustices, developing responsibility, co-operating and working to prevent future inequities, and confirming both in the roles of father and son.

Case 3E: Persecution[7]

March, 1993: Sergei, 23 years, a storeman and part-time pugilist, who had attended weekly therapy for several months, told me of his continuing confusion and lack of confidence in his social life. An immigrant from the former Soviet Union, he had come with his family to Melbourne in 1988. Sergei described himself as having been shy and a loner since childhood and he remembered many moments of torment when his school mates in Moscow had chased him home from classes whilst calling out: 'Jid! Jid!' (a common anti-semitic insult) and beating him up whenever they had caught him. Shortly after arriving in Australia, Sergei had commenced training in boxing to learn how to defend himself and boost his self-image. This had partly worked but he said that he was still troubled by self doubt and indecision: Should he go ahead and marry his fiancee, Nina, 20, a cosmetician? When should he assert himself in public? Sergei even had fancies of standing up in a tram one day and punching the ticket collector 'just for the heck of it, to feel more of a man!'.

At this particular therapy session, Sergei was especially irritated by an acquaintance, Maurice, 28, who had propositioned Nina. Sergei had ended the friendship with Maurice but felt that any unpleasantness that remained between them whenever they met in their social group was due to his own fault. 'How can I get this feeling out of my head that I am to blame?' queried Sergei. 'I would like to feel that I am right and Maurice is wrong but I always feel that, when anything goes wrong, I am in the wrong'. 'It sounds as if you have a saboteur inside you', I commented, 'a persecutor who makes you feel less of a man. What does your saboteur tell you to destroy your confidence?'

---

7   This case was originally presented in the 'General Practitioner', *Adis International 2*, 9, May 1994, 9–10.

'I don't know', replied Sergei, stopping his self-recriminations and appearing intrigued by this idea. 'Yet there are many areas in which you are competent', I continued, 'You got out of bed this morning without breaking a leg. You ate breakfast without staining your clothes. You have recently passed your nursing aid's examinations with credit. If you are confident in these areas, you can learn to be confident in relationships, to have your needs met. I wonder how your saboteur invites you to forget that you are basically a confident guy?' Sergei remained silent and thoughtful, so I ventured further with our conversation: 'I wonder if your saboteur, your internal persecutor, tells you that you have no rights in this, or any other matter. Certainly, you learnt early enough from your persecuting schoolmates that you were considered to have no rights to safety, comfort and freedom from fear. Your saboteur seems to tell you that you have to take it on the chin. What would happen if you stepped into the ring with your boxing gloves on, facing your saboteur as an opponent? Would you take it on the chin or would you K. O. the saboteur? Would you write a letter to your saboteur, delivering a K. O. blow, telling your saboteur that you do have rights?' We had come to the end of our conversation for that moment. Sergei, agreeing to bring his letter to our next meeting, stood up and gave me a firm handshake. 'This was a good session', he said briskly, 'a very good session!'

Sergei's conversation with his persecutor:

SERGEI: Should I go out and talk to some girls tomorrow?

SABOTEUR: No, it is too hard. They would not like you.

SERGEI: But I am not bad looking, good body.

SABOTEUR: Good body has nothing to do with it, they will think you are uninteresting.

SERGEI: But I can be interesting when I am not afraid of people.

SABOTEUR: Yep, that's the point. You won't be able to fight your fears and, being afraid, you would block all your thought processes. So you will not have anything to say.

SERGEI: But I am supposed to try anyway. Because if I do not, I will never respect myself.

SABOTEUR: Go ahead. Find out what it is like to feel humiliated and embarrassed. You think you can handle it but in your mind things always appear to be smoother and easier. Experience the dreadful reality.

(Following this, Sergei told a fellow student, who asked him if he was of the Russian Orthodox Faith, that he was Jewish, a fact which Sergei had always kept hidden in public).

Discussion

The 'developmental map' can be considered the therapeutic context used within which Sergei examines the diffidence that has troubled him since his youth. Sergei used many words which enabled me to imagine the real of his world: confusion, lack of confidence, shy, a loner, many moments of torment. Sergei appeared to regard himself within an I–It position as 'weak and ineffectual'. I believe that Sergei and I were able to achieve mutuality within an I–Thou position and to be included within the therapeutic conversation, not only because of the Jewish kinship (and perhaps Russian ancestry) that we shared but because of my own experiences of persecution in primary school in the 1950s: I had a lisp and wore corrective footwear, I wore glasses and was nick-named 'Four-eyes' and Gunzburg often became 'Gunzbum!'. Because I suffered repeated ear infections and wore a rubber cap over my head to protect my ears when swimming, I was teased as 'a sissy girl'. So I was well able to imagine the real of Sergei's persecution! Note how Sergei fantasized acting out his aggression against the tram conductor. He can be regarded as attempting to reconcile the contrary: persecutor/persecuted, by becoming the persecutor. By using a metaphor within his field of interest: boxing, I encouraged him to explore other ways that he could counter his sense of helplessness which remained since his persecution during his schooling. Persecutor/survivor of persecution is also a contrary which can be reconciled successfully in contesting the persecution. In writing a letter to his saboteur and discovering a non-aggressive means to contest his persecution, Sergei can be considered as confirming himself as a competent client and I can be regarded as confirming myself as a competent therapist. Client/therapist can be viewed as another contrary to be reconciled during the therapeutic conversation.

Case 3F: Embarrassment[8]

November, 1993: Gregory, 26 years, a biochemist, was telling me about his despair over the end of a nine-year relationship with Bill, 40, a year earlier. Bill had proven to be a compulsive liar and repeatedly unfaithful and had embarrassed Gregory to no end with his larrikin remarks and behaviour in

---

8   This case was originally presented in the 'General Practitioner', *Adis International 2*, 14, August 1994, 23.

public throughout the duration of the friendship. Two months after the separation, Gregory had met Greg, 30, a counsellor, and, although this intimacy was progressing well, Gregory would become angry whenever Greg joked around within their social group. Gregory had been particularly irritated when, on the previous Sunday, Greg had toyed around with the sugar bowl and spoon at a restaurant. Gregory related how he had been teased mercilessly at school during his adolescence for 'not doing all the things that most boys do', that is sport, dating girls, fighting his schoolmates, etc. I invited Gregory to consider whether part of his reaction to Greg's practical joking was due to the disparagement that he had experienced as a teenager: 'Perhaps the jeering of your school mates encouraged you to want to be inconspicuous?', I queried, 'yet, first Bill, and now Greg, have a knack of drawing all the attention in a crowd towards you and themselves with their high jinks. I guess you are most comfortable when you are the invisible man. How can you be imperceptible with those two around you?' 'That's it!' Gregory exclaimed excitedly, sitting up in his chair, enlivened, 'You have hit the nail on the head. I had not thought of it like that before. I cannot hide when I am with them'. Gregory's depression lifted and he appeared to tolerate Greg's buffoonery with more equanimity. Our conversation moved on to assertiveness. How could Gregory counter the barbs of prejudiced and insensitive people whenever he encountered them?

Discussion

The 'developmental and systemic maps' can be regarded as the therapeutic contexts in which Gregory explored his behaviour: how he first learnt to experience his embarrassment and the circumstances in which he experienced it currently. Some of Gregory's words that enabled the therapist to imagine the real of his world were: despair, embarrassed, compulsive liar, repeatedly unfaithful, being jeered at for not doing all the things that most boys do. Gregory appeared to blame himself (within an I–It position) as incompetent within intimate relationships because he felt 'bad' at certain times when in the company of Bill and Greg. I highlighted that perhaps at certain times Gregory felt shame because he had been shamed by school-mates who had treated him adversely (within an I–It position), mocking his homosexuality and that perhaps he had wanted to withdraw all his life from contact with others for fear of continued teasing. Bill, with his constant lying and infidelities, certainly appeared to have disacknowledged Gregory in a similar manner to the schoolyard tormentors. But I was not so certain that this was the situation with Greg. Rather, the jovial nature of his current partner did not allow Gregory to remain hidden. This statement can be considered as attempting to reconcile the contraries: identity/identity diffusion and intimacy/isolation. Rather than having developed a definite sense of self, Gregory appeared to have wanted to remain invisible, to disappear into the crowd. Rather than join with Greg as an intimate partner, and grow with him, Gregory appeared to have wanted Greg to remain inconspicuous with him. This is a very common circumstance with survivors of abuse. Perhaps the best way to contest our abusers, however, is to develop our resources and overcome the effects of their abuse. Indeed, the best revenge may be to have a good life! Gregory seemed to grasp this idea with enthusiasm and therapy appeared to enable him to confirm his ability as an assertive person. My statement can also be regarded as an act of inclusion, drawing Gregory into a conversation, within an I–Thou position, about embarrassment. Most therapists and clients, I believe, need to deal with situations of being derided by others at times in their lives.

Case 3G: The courage to become[9]

February, 1993: Karen, 23 years, unemployed, was telling me of her aspirations. She had wanted to leave home within the past year but lack of assets and income had made renting a flat an impossibility. Her mother, Rosa, 57, had always stressed that Karen should leave the family following a wedding breakfast. Over the previous twelve months, Karen had looked for employment but the economic recession, together with her obesity, made it unlikely that she would acquire a job in the near future. Karen had preferred a vocation in the hospitality industry, but, as Karen said, 'they don't favour fat waitresses!'. Karen said that she was becoming bored and despairing of ever finding work.

Karen proceeded to tell me her story during a series of fortnightly sessions over the next ten months. She did not reveal to her family that she was seeking the help of a therapist for fear of them calling her 'stupid'. Ever since she was a toddler, Karen could remember her father calling her stupid. She described the father, Alan, 59, an invalid pensioner for the past eight years due to a 'nervous breakdown', as a misogynist. Karen's three elder brothers appeared to have copied the pattern of disparaging their mother and sister from their father. Karen listed her interests as: light classical music, detective novels, a variety of styles in food and romantic films. Once every week she played tennis with Andrew, 28, a neighbour and student of French polishing. We discussed an episode that had occurred when Karen was about six years old, when a man in the park had exposed his genitals to her. Karen wondered

---

9   This case was originally presented in the 'General Practitioner', *Adis International 2*, 14, August 1994, 23.

if she had been frightened of sexual relationships since then. She said that she had never had a boyfriend and wondered if she carried the extra weight on her body to present herself as less attractive. In doing so, she would not have to worry about how to handle the approaches of men who might be interested in her. I asked Karen if she would write a description of the incident in the park. Karen wrote:

> It was a bright and sunny day. I was happily playing at the park with a little girl whose name I never knew. Then came a man, a man I thought I knew, who changed all that happiness to sadness. After seeing him I felt very empty, confused and scared. I did not know what to do so I put it out of my mind.

I told Karen that I was touched by the simple poignancy of her essay: the account of a young child being frightened away from the joys that adulthood can bring by a man who had carelessly and irresponsibly dumped his emotional problems onto Karen and her young friend. I also shared with Karen my thoughts that there might be another factor operating here. I wondered if Rosa had invited Karen, at an early age, to be her partner against the apparent patriarchal attitudes of the men in the family? The assault by the man in the park might have convinced the young Karen that she needed to be an ally with her mother against the assaults of men, both inside and outside her family. The men in her family had devalued their womenfolk constantly. I wondered if Rosa had written a script for Karen, one of helplessness, one that reflected Rosa's helplessness? What would have to happen for Karen to retire from this role of being Rosa's partner against the oppression of women by men and for Karen to write her own script? I felt that Rosa had taught Karen courage at one level: the determination to withstand the tyranny of her menfolk and work towards family cohesion, doing as best she could in difficult circumstances. What would have to happen for Karen to find the courage to become her own person? perhaps to leave the family territory and fight the oppression on her own terms? I asked Karen to list some ways of reaching out to the world outside her family and to imagine what her life might be like in five years time. Karen wrote:

> Ten ways to contact the world:
> 1. Going for a drive
> 2. Going for walks
> 3. Writing letters to friends
> 4. Talking to neighbours
> 5. Reading a book

6. Thinking about the future

7. Listening to music

8. Window shopping

9. Going to the movies

10. Looking after a baby

What life will be like in five years:

Life will be fantastic. In five years I will be a very successful career woman who is on the verge of starting her own successful business and has a husband and children who love and support her in all she does'.

A fortnight later, Karen told me that Rosa had introduced Milos, 40, to Karen as a marriage proposition. Karen had sat down with her mother and pointed out that Milos was an unemployed invalid, with one hundred dollars in the bank, who said that he was waiting for his mother to die and leave him her house. Rosa had appeared to listen to Karen's assessment of the situation respectfully and had ceased her pressure to make a match. Karen had invited Andrew out to a cousin's wedding, something that she would have never contemplated doing a year previously. And she was buying a new wardrobe because all her current clothes were getting too big for her!

Discussion

The 'developmental, feminist and systemic maps' can be regarded as the therapeutic contexts within which Karen explored how she was first abused by men during her childhood, the patriarchal themes underlying the abusers' behaviour and how her mother may have enlisted Karen as a support in the mother's struggles with the men in the family. Some words that Karen used which enabled the therapist to imagine the real of her world were: fat, bored, despairing, stupid, sadness, empty, confused, scared. Karen seemed to have learnt early, from her father and brothers and the sexual abuser in the park, that women are there to be the repository for men's negative feelings, to be dumped on and bear the brunt of male aggression. These men can certainly be considered as treating Karen (and Rosa) within an I–It position. Rosa, however, also appeared to regard Karen within an I–It position: the daughter was to give the mother help against the inequity within the family, with scant consideration for the daughter's needs. Karen's account of the abuse, and her lists for the future, can be regarded as acts of inclusion: therapists and clients both, I believe, need to contest the various abuses within the community.

They also need to consider ways to achieve their future potential and independence, yet retain their connectedness with others. Intimacy/isolation can be regarded as a contrary which Karen reconciled. Her male abusers created an environment for Karen in which she felt inferior and isolated yet, in her list of ways to connect with the world, Karen details how she might make contact. Karen's refusal of marriage to Milos and her inviting Andrew to the family wedding can be considered acts whereby she is confirming her freedom of choice, exploring her own directions towards intimacy.

Case 3H: Artistic block

December, 1993: Daniel, 28 years, an employee in the catering/ hospitality area until he developed chronic fatigue syndrome several months earlier, told me how he had experienced artistic block for many years. He had been a painter, favouring pastels and charcoal as his media, until his early twenties when his creative drive had ceased and he had taken to drinking spirits for solace. Daniel had joined Alcoholics Anonymous two years previously and had been sober for the past five months. Over the previous few weeks, Daniel had taken up painting again and had found that this activity had revived some fairly powerful memories and emotions from his past.

Daniel related how his stepbrother, Dieter, now 43, had sexually abused him between the ages of three and ten. Dieter would have been eighteen years old when he had commenced violating Daniel and we discussed the abuse of power inherent within such a situation. I asked Daniel if he would write a letter to Dieter contesting his abuse. Daniel wrote his essay and shared it with me at our next weekly meeting:

> I have been lying in bed sleepless over the past several nights wondering if there is anything that I could say or do that would change the way I feel about the way you treated me. All I can say at this point is that I do not blame you, or hold you responsible (for my future recovery) but that what you did was so terribly, absolutely wrong.

Daniel described how Dieter had taken him onto a raft, floating out to sea out of Daniel's depth, when he was seven years old and how Dieter had rubbed his genitals against Daniel's body. Dieter had also been practising anal intercourse on Daniel since he was a toddler and Daniel related an incident when he had wanted to go to the toilet to empty his bowels and Dieter had been lying in wait for him. Dieter had followed him into the toilet and had penetrated him. Daniel had envisaged 'a mess everywhere' and had burst into tears.

Dieter had attempted to abuse Daniel's younger brother who had told his mother of Dieter's actions. The mother had asked Daniel if Dieter had abused Daniel and Daniel denied it, for fear of Dieter going to prison. Dieter had ceased abusing Daniel after this incident. Daniel commented that he had first remembered the scene on the raft two years ago when Ted, 52, Daniel's sponsor at Alcoholics Anonymous, whom Daniel was supposed to telephone whenever he felt the urge to drink, propositioned him and they had commenced a sexual intimacy. 'I think that your Unconscious is very clever', I responded softly, 'I think that your Unconscious signals to you when you are being exploited by others'.

We discussed Daniel's feelings of when Dieter had abused him on the raft, feelings of being trapped and terror of being pushed into the water and drowning, and when Dieter had completely ignored Daniel's needs to use the toilet, wanting only his own selfish gratification. This had been a totally cruel and inappropriate use of Daniel's body, a veritable rape with Daniel wanting to expel his wastes and Dieter pushing them back into him. I asked if Daniel felt that Dieter had poisoned him in this manner. Daniel replied that, much of the time, he did feel as if he was filled with excreta.

Daniel had recalled the incident on the raft when Ted wanted to exploit Daniel for his own pleasure, when Ted's role was to protect and nurture Daniel from the urge to become inebriated. Like Dieter, Ted had betrayed Daniel's trust but Daniel's Unconscious had been an 'effective friend' and had warned Daniel not to continue his relationship with Ted. When Ted had invited Daniel to move in with him, Daniel had declined. 'Therapy can train your Unconscious to continue to be your companion,' I commented, 'alerting you against the attempted violations of others'. Daniel handed me another note that he had written: 'It's not the sex (with Ted) that bothered me. It was the betrayal which has led to my current mistrust and fear of intimacy'. I shared with Daniel the following story of how my Unconscious comes to my aid.

Case 3H: (i) The Ice Queen
October, 1992: Gerda, 22 years, a deferred economics/politics student, was bothered by her relationships. Her boyfriends, of which there was no shortage – possibly due to Gerda's stunning beauty, always seemed to end their relationships complaining that she was aloof and unaffectionate. 'They call me the Ice Queen', Gerda said, 'but I feel comfortable in keeping my distance. I am not interested in an immediate physical relationship. The guys all think that because I am a blue-eyed blonde model-type, that I must be hot stuff in bed! I want to be sure that they are attracted to me for qualities

other than just my looks. Is that so wrong?'. Gerda said that it was important for her to sort out the closeness-distance arrangements in her friendships because she was planning a trip to Europe in five months and wanted to enjoy it to the full, without any harassment.

Gerda told me about the many violations within her family of origin. She had little reason to trust the men in her life. Her alcohol-abusing father, Martin, 52, had left her mother, Leila, 48, whom he had physically mistreated for many years, when Gerda was eight. Her elder brother, Thomas, 30, had sexually abused Gerda between the ages of four and twelve. Her adolescence, she said, had been a disaster area. Gerda had been shy, hesitant and frightened of approaching her peers and, although she had gained confidence during her years of tertiary study and now enjoyed social intercourse, she still did not warm readily to deeper intimacies. Gerda had become depressed towards the end of the previous year and had chosen to defer her studies for a year and spend some time overseas.

We talked for a while about how maintaining her distance enabled Gerda to protect her 'personal territory'. She had developed a number of assertive statements that were cool yet courteous. At the end of our session, Gerda said that she had valued the opportunity to talk about her troubled feelings. She decided that she was perfectly happy keeping her contacts conversational and that, for the present, she would continue the role of Ice Queen which kept her safe. That night I dreamt of a blue and white striped flag with a white cross on a blue square in one corner. I consulted my Encyclopaedia Britannica, discovered that the flag which I had seen in my dream was Greek and laughed softly. During therapy, Gerda and I had talked about her planned holiday to the Greek Isles. I said that I had visited the Acropolis three years previously. I guess that, secretly, I wished that I might join Gerda during her travels. My dream had signalled my hidden attraction towards Gerda. It is absolutely essential for therapists to be aware of unconscious desires for their clients and never to act them out. (One of my feminist colleagues commented when I shared this story with her: 'But would you have been dreaming of Gerda, John, if she had not been so physically beautiful?')

We spent the rest of our meeting discussing how Dieter, Ted and Gerda's abusers appeared to have demanded their 'patriarchal privileges'. Dieter and Ted could both be considered caretakers to Daniel, at various stages of his life, yet they had ignored Daniel's needs for safety and nurturance to pursue their own gratification, as had Gerda's father and elder brother. Her boyfriends appeared only to respond to their physical attraction towards her, discounting her when she was reluctant to accede to their wishes. Daniel related how, recently, at a New Year's Eve party, he had been tempted to 'get stuck into the grog' but had restricted himself to four glasses of lemonade. I shook Daniel's hand and remarked that I thought that 'this was gold medal stuff', a real achievement. For the first time, Daniel's solemn face cracked a smile from ear to ear.

Discussion

The 'developmental, psychodynamic systemic and feminist maps' can be considered the therapeutic context of Daniel's struggles: how Dieter had abused Daniel during his childhood and how Ted had continued the pattern of abuse during Daniel's adulthood and how both abusers appeared to have followed patriarchal scripts. Some of Daniel's words which enabled the therapist to imagine the real of his world were: chronic fatigue, artistic block, drinking spirits for solace, filled with excreta, betrayal, mistrust, fear of intimacy. Dieter and Ted can certainly be regarded as relating to Daniel within an I–It position: Daniel was simply a sexual thing for their pleasure. Telling Daniel the story of Gerda can be considered an act of inclusion: I believe that therapists and clients both need to be aware of how their Unconscious can be usefully tapped within their lives. Three contraries can be considered to have been reconciled within this therapeutic conversation:

1. Basic mistrust/trust and intimacy/isolation – inviting Daniel into a genuine dialogue, within an I–Thou position, in which he can experience trust in a non-exploitative relationship with a male therapist.

2. Industry/inferiority and generativity/stagnation – encouraging Daniel to continue to use his artistic skills to develop his sense of confidence and progress forward in his life.

3. Unconscious/ conscious – using unconscious resources (validating the memories of his abuses) to overcome conscious emotional struggles (grieving, letting go and successfully contesting the abuses). My handshake can be regarded as an effective way to confirm Daniel's ability to care for himself adequately.

Case 31: Lifting the fog

November, 1994: Sue, 38 years, a nurse, was describing the fears and episodes of panic that had erupted through her calm exterior for many years. These episodes had become worse over the past few months and, indeed, had influenced Sue to walk out of a family therapy session with Simon, another therapist, the previous week. Sue and her family were attending family therapy to address their elder son's reticence to do his schoolwork and his apparent lack of hope for the future. Simon knew that I had counselled Sue individually for some time and that she still occasionally saw me to get a different angle on an aspect of her life. With Sue and the family's permission, Simon and I had shared our thoughts as to how we saw our respective roles in helping the family as a whole.

One of the issues that Sue had felt comfortable to share only with me was an episode of childhood sexual abuse when Sue was about four, when an adult family friend had taken her for a bike ride and had placed her hand on his genitals. Sue felt that, although this had startled and confused her, there was more there 'hidden in the mist' that was troubling her. Sue thought that there might have been other abuses perpetrated about which she had forgotten and about which she might need to remember. I knew that Sue enjoyed writing and asked her if she would compose an account of her feelings. Sue wrote:

> Hovering around, obscuring the picture from her, the cloud enveloped all that she did. She operated in a strange, delicate way, trying at times to see into the far distance, both past and future. The present would not allow this fog to lift. All around her was a quietness, a stillness which somehow allowed the tinkling sounds of the past to filter through the all-enveloping mist.

> The sounds brought fear to the surface of her mind. Her body responded with a quickened heartbeat and short gasping breaths followed by long, deep sighs. What could it be? Sometimes she thought that perhaps it was a family abuse. Not a physical abuse, more an emotional abuse. Her family. A strange family this one. They operated in a twilight world of make-believe. Make believe that everything is all right. Make believe that these 'nasty' emotions weren't there. Even as she tried to grasp the notion of abuse, it slipped through her fingers like water, not being able to form its true pattern as the container had no true shape. Abuse. A hard, short opening sound with a soft subtle intonation on the end. Connotations of short sharp action followed by softly smothered cries of pain. Dictionary definitions are of no use here she thought, as she tried to pin it down, put a name to it and put it on the shelf with all the other hurts. The words are the clues. They come and go but on reflection, if you hold them long enough the feeling grows that something happened once, long ago. Fear, pain deep inside, somebody hold me, lost in the night. She wandered on down the dusty, tree-lined street, warm dust on bare feet, toes and feet kicking up dust in the shifting mist around her.

Sometimes she thought that although the path twisted and turned in an endless fashion, it must lead to a pivotal point where all was clear and calm. The calmness of a gently lapping sea against a creamy white sand. It was a fear of the unknown which seemed to startle her at unexpected moments.

There was no sense to it, no logic in these feelings. It wasn't as if these sensed abuses had a place or a time or even a name with which they could be classified, sorted and labeled.

It became a mist of uncertainty which was difficult to deal with. How can something sensed become encoded in reality?

The journey down that dusty road continued. Occasionally the enveloping mist lifted a little, the fear subsided and the heart settled into an easy rhythm. Always there, lurking in some corner of her mind was the unexplained 'thing'.

As she trudged along, deep in thought, she felt again that sensation of heat, dust and dry air. Whatever it was, it belonged to that once-upon-a-time, a-long-time-ago place in her past when she lived in that border country town.

There was a river there. It flowed fast and strong along one edge of the town. It provided a border across which she hardly ever crossed as that road led to the unknown places. An old wooden bridge crossed the river. As cars crossed over, you could hear the twang of tyres hitting the loose boards and the rumble as they sped past. Once she remembered driving along beside the river with her father. She saw on the other side of the river a camp of higgeldy-piggeldy makeshift huts and houses. She asked her father what it was. He said that is where the aborigines live. She remembered feeling shocked and sad. She had lived in that town for some time and had not known of this place on the edge of her world.

As she walked along the river bank she began to sense an atmosphere of sadness and horror. Disquiet at the sensed but unseen began to impinge on her awareness of her surroundings. The sensed disquiet began to grow.

She remembered the clear-cut images of early childhood. Warm dry air, dust picked up and blown along straight dry roads. Heat and dust, warmth from the sun. Although the atmosphere was dry and the sun had a strength to it, the street she lived in provided a shaded haven from the harsh world outside its environs.

The street had no footpaths, just a dusty dry road with grass verges and tall umbrella-like trees. The feeling of turning the corner from the harsh outside heat into the tunnel of coolness and shade. Kicking the dust, feeling its cooling ooze through her toes.

At the end of the long road was a wire fence with a gate which always stood open. Once, in that long-ago place, her sisters took her through the gate to an open area covered in yellow daisies. They sat and together made daisy chains which they strung around their necks, around the pusher in which she sat joyfully trundled home to show the mother.

It was beginning to become clearer now. The mist lifting, shifting slightly, now giving glimpses of the way ahead.

One day, as the sense of unease began to grow beyond the point of despair, all became clear. The unacknowledged feelings, unspoken fears and terrors erupted. The cry came from somewhere deep inside, travelling from the past, erupting into a howl of horror. Somewhere a soul was extinguished in a violent apocalyptic fashion.

She remembered now. It was the mother who cried out like that. It was the mother whose anguish could not bear the silence after the spoken words. The child was frightened. This sound she had not heard before. This enraged cry at loss.

Somehow that cry signalled the beginning of the walk, the journey down the dusty road to the dark house where not much light came, of waiting in that house on that Sunday before Easter for her father to come and take her home, of not wanting to go home because something horrifying in its suddenness had happened. The fear of the unknown began then. The child's world irrevocably changed when her sister died. The feelings of aloneness, of separation. Each family member trying to come to grips with the tragedy in the separate silences which could not be breached. The child just wanted to be hugged, to be held and comforted. Somehow the family retreated, too damaged, too hurt to repair the fundamental damage done by silence. They blocked out the bad things, pretended they weren't there. On the surface, pretence at normality of life going on but ignoring always the reality of what was happening around them. Not able to move away from the twilight world of fiction.

After sharing her essay with me, Sue was more able to discuss her family's reaction to her sister's death in a motor vehicle accident when Sue was eight years old. Sue had mentioned this event briefly during our initial meeting some years ago and had never returned to the subject. We considered how the family 'closed up', offered no emotional support to each other and proceeded with their lives as if nothing untoward had happened. From that moment, Sue had learnt not to seek support for her own needs. I was able to tell Sue of my own arduous journey through a fog of eroticism and frustration.

Case 31: (i) Healing through meeting

I had struggled for many years to avoid sexualizing the many women whom I met on the way and a few men also. At various times, I had been diagnosed 'manic-depressive', 'hypomanic' and 'suffering a personality disorder', and had been prescribed medication which had proved somewhat calming though it had not alleviated my internal sexual strivings. When, during mid-life, I began to develop 'the hots' for young boys, I thought it appropriate to seek help from a practitioner skilled in both individual and family psychotherapy. After many months of weekly meetings, my therapist suggested tentatively: 'John, it sounds as if at some stage in your early life you were the focus of another person's sexual activity'. I remember responding to this statement with an enormous sigh of relief: 'At last, someone has mentioned the unmentionable!'. I was able to divulge some early memories, that had surfaced during therapy, and that had bothered me for weeks: shadowy images of me lying in a crib and a man's face hovering above me; a man's mouth on a toddler's genitals and an unleashing of sensations. I had always thought it might have been my maternal grandfather who was the perpetrator (he had been imprisoned in Buchenwald concentration camp and came out of that experience mentally unstable). I never solved the mystery of who the perpetrator was, within therapy, but validating the experiences of sexual abuse certainly helped me to restrain my tussles with the demons within and my attraction towards young boys dissipated. Indeed, I appeared more able to channel my sexual conflicts into my writing. During a visit to my parents in Perth, Western Australia, some years later, I told my mother of my experiences of sexual abuse that I had recalled during therapy. Mother's first reaction was: 'I did not know that this was happening'. I was quick to assure her that I was not blaming her, or indeed anyone, but wondered if she might help me fit the jigsaw together. Mother thought for a few moments and continued: 'It was definitely not your grandfather. You and he were very chummy together and he would not have harmed you in this way. I do think I know who it was though. We had a young labourer on the chicken farm at Gosnells in the early days. He was a strange fellow, very dogmatic in his opinions and beliefs. He was with us for eighteen months. Then we let him go because we felt uneasy about several episodes of unreliability and lying. There was certainly every opportunity for him to molest you behind our backs'. I gave Mother a hug! 'Who knows what the truth of the matter is?' I commented to Sue, 'but the fact that my mother took me seriously, and sat with me to tend to my needs to talk about it, was very healing'.

We talked about the feminist attitudes towards sexual violation; how the abusers, who were usually men, could be regarded as considering themselves 'entitled to their male rights for easy gratification'. As therapy progressed, Sue started asking more from her emotionally aloof husband and her sons, both in their family therapy with Simon and at home. Recently, Sue sent me the following inscription on a card bearing the illustration of Vincent van Gogh's painting *First Steps*:

> To my friend, Dr Gunzburg,
>
> This is just to say thank you for your care, comfort and consideration of me over the past months. It is only now, that I realize that I was being 'looked after' when I was set on the path to your door. Thank you for the stories and the hugs and the books you lent me. I realize that in some ways, The Journey is just beginning but I now hope the paths I am choosing will be the best ones for me.
>
> Until we meet again 'May God hold you in the hollow of His hand',
>
> Yours sincerely, Sue.

Discussion

The 'developmental and feminist maps' can be considered the therapeutic context within which Sue and I discussed the evolution of our struggles and the nature of the actions of our abusers. Our resolution through creative writing can be regarded as being grounded within the 'spiritual map'. Some of the words that Sue used that enabled me to imagine the real of her world were: fears, panic, startled, confused, quietness, stillness, enveloping mist, short gasping breaths, long deep sighs. Some of the words I used so that Sue could imagine the real of my world were: fog, eroticism, frustration, sexual strivings, manic-depression, personality disorder. Our abusers can be considered as viewing us within an I–It position: Sue and I being regarded as things for their sexual gratification rather than children who required protection and nurturance. Sue's family, at the time of the sister's death, can also be considered as viewing themselves within an I–It position: needing to get on with their lives, in robotic fashion, without tending to their needs to grieve and comfort each other. This can be regarded as an example of what Buber might call mismeeting. Writing her essay, and my telling Sue my story, can be considered acts of inclusion: I believe that we all need to be understood, accept losses, grieve, let go, move on. Sue appeared more able to ask me for space to speak her grief for missed opportunities within her family of origin and be able to ask for her needs to be met within her current family and to be acknowledged more. For both Sue and I, the contraries that can be considered reconciled were: identity/ identity diffusion, intimacy/isolation, generativity/stagnation and ego-integrity/despair. We can be regarded as finding ourselves and being able to name our abuse through our writing, connecting more effectively with each other and other intimates within our families, and moving past our emotional struggles towards a greater sense of inner peace and fulfillment. This therapy can be regarded as confirming both Sue and I as successful participants within the therapeutic conversation and as creative survivors and contesters of abuse.

Case 3J: The homicidal lesbian terrorist
December, 1993: Annie, 25 years, unemployed, was telling me of the fury that had raged within her for most of her life. The child of a rape of her mother, Shirl, now 49, by the mother's stepfather, Brian, now 79, Annie had also been sexually abused by Brian when she was eight years old. Annie said that Shirl had neglected and physically abused her daughter for much of Annie's life and she had left home at sixteen years of age to live on the streets. Annie had become involved within the drug scene and, two years previously, had entered a rehabilitation centre. Annie had had a number of lovers and was grieving the end of her last one-and-a-half year intimacy with Fay, 25, four months ago. Annie described Fay as the 'quiet, vengeful' type and had found herself getting angrier and angrier and wanting to do Fay physical violence. Annie had walked away from the friendship because of this. I asked Annie if she would write a letter to Brian contesting his rapes of both Shirl and Annie, and to Shirl contesting her emotional and physical abuses of Annie.

A month passed and much of New South Wales had been engulfed in flames, most of the bush fires having been started by arsonists. Annie came to our next session sporting a T-shirt which bore the words 'I can't even think STRAIGHT!' and said that she had been 'raging within' since our last session, though she had not acted out her anger either physically or in renewed reliance on drugs or alcohol. Annie showed me an essay on her anger and two letters that she had written to Shirl:

Anger

I get so god-damned angry about men past and present, that so-called power makes them so stupid. All they do is spend hate in any way possible.

All this bushfires stuff shits me. Some man lit the fires then the news is crapping on about the firemen. What about all the women helping? No, it's men, men.

From now on any man that talks shit to me is going to get clobbered. I'm not going to let anyone ride over me. If anyone says shit to me they either get educated fast or get ditched. It's my way or the highway.

I'm still pissed off with Fay. I get pissed off about having to do everything myself. I'm pissed off about being a target because I am myself.

I am sick of the way women are treated publicly.

I hate straight people, especially the ones who say that they're gay-friendly but still put down gays.

Hets [heterosexuals] are fucked.

Dear Shirl Jones,

Thanks for the time(s) you:
1. left me in hospital for two weeks on my own when I was born.
2. left me to play by myself unguarded.
3. let your boyfriend Jim hold me to ridicule, boss me, push me around. He wasn't my father.
4. beat me because the police brought me home for my own safety, or when I was finding it hard with schoolwork, or I stole Jim's money to get back at you/him, or when I ran away from home, lied, was late.
5. whacked my hands ten or more times with rulers, but I learnt not to cry, or flinch, just to spite you.
6. beat me with your fists, and kicked me in the ribs so hard I couldn't breathe, and then ordered me to do the dishes at the same time.
7. did not let me have a pet. Every time I got one you took it away, because you said children can't look after them for long,

because of children's short attention-span. All children you
saw did this, so I was a child, so I was going to do it too.

8. said I could have a proper birthday or Xmas party but I never
    did.

9. were either a bad role model or not one at all.

10. did not encourage me when I needed it.

11. put me down every time about my relationships, lifestyle,
    career, emotion, health, being fat, a smoker, a drinker, a
    lesbian, my mistakes.

12. did not support me once in my life.

13. criticized my friends, lovers, choices, pets, haircuts, clothes.

14. never praised me, just for the sake of it.

15. ignored me, pushing me into the background, especially when
    you had boyfriends.

16. lied, and told me bullshit about people, the world and life.

17. threatened and taunted me.

18. made my life a misery, and then laughed at me when I went to
    get professional help or pretended that I was making it all up,
    saying it's in my head or that I'm doing it to spite you.

THANK YOU MOTHER

Dear Miss Shirl Jones,

I wish to notify you of the following information. That I, formerly
Annie Jessica Jones, do not wish to be related to you in any form
whatsoever. I do not wish to be contacted by you except via a legal
representative. I do not wish you to personally come near me, my
home, pets or friends. I am prepared to take legal action if this arises.
In return this is the last time I contact you or your mother personally.
If you wish to contest this notice then contact me through your legal
representative,

SEE YOU IN HELL,

Yours Sincerely, etc.

We discussed Annie's restraints. Here was the fury writhing inside her yet
she said that she had been involved in only two episodes of physical violence
with Fay and had preferred to distance herself from the friendship rather
than commit another assault. In this regard, Annie certainly had bettered
Shirl – who appeared to have enacted out her own rage continually on her

daughter. I expressed my admiration of Annie in that it was obvious to me that our last meeting had stirred up some pretty powerful emotions for her yet she had kept a lid on her temper, avoiding any self-destructive acts or violence towards other people. Annie's anger seemed primarily directed towards Shirl for the nurturing and protection that she had denied Annie during her growing years. There was no question in my mind that Shirl's abuse of Annie was absolutely wrong. Yet I commented aloud that I could not help wondering how much of Shirl's behaviour had been influenced by Brian's criminal irresponsibility. Many men considered themselves entitled to their 'male rights' and appeared to enjoy abusing power to get these 'male rights' met. Annie was certainly angry at men and, indeed, all her struggles had been grounded within the relationships of her heterosexual caretakers; Shirl, Jim and Shirl's other boyfriends. I could understand how Annie experienced the straight world as inherently evil so I shared the following story with her:

Case 3J: (i) Life stinks!

June, 1991: Nasa, 30 years, an office worker, was broken-hearted about the death of her four months old daughter Amira several weeks previously. The babe had succumbed to Hoffman's disease, a type of congenital muscular dystrophy. Nasa's chances of having another infant afflicted with the same disease was 25 per cent and she and her husband, Tony, 31, a bricklayer, had decided not to have more children until a definite pre-natal test had been developed to detect whether her foetus was affected or not. Nasa had been told that such a test was about two years away.

We spent three or four weekly therapy sessions discussing Nasa's sadness. She was finding it difficult to get back into her work routine and Nasa said that she was experiencing envy that so many of her friends were commencing their families, whereas she and Tony had been frustrated in their plans. Nasa showed me a photograph of Amira, a sweet-faced child, and said that she and her mother visited the grave regularly on weekends to place flowers there. She said that Tony was a lovely husband and a wonderful comfort to her. 'Am I a real mother?', Nasa asked, 'I am forgetting so much about Amira now that she is gone. But I still have the stretch marks on my body to show that I was pregnant with her. It is not fair that I have lost my shape and have no baby to show for it. I don't know if I am a real mother'.

We discussed how, though memories of detailed images often fade with time after loss, the feelings that we enjoyed during those good moments with the deceased often remained. I asked Nasa to contemplate, and perhaps list, the warm times that she had remembered with Amira. Nasa liked music. I asked her to listen to Beethoven's *Pastoral* Symphony, No. 6, with its pleasant depiction of country life, stormy crisis and spiritual hymn of healing that concluded the work. Nasa's sadness lifted, her energy returned, she became more absorbed in her work and social life and, at our fifth meeting, commented: 'I visited the paediatrician who cared for Amira during her final illness last week. He has been kind and decent to me throughout and wanted to know how I was coping. I liked what he said to me. I said that I was going OK, but that life stinks! He replied: No. Hoffman's disease stinks!'.

'I think there is a bit of a similarity in Nasa's situation to yours', I suggested to Annie, 'Hets don't stink. Abusive Hets stink!'. 'In fact', I said, 'in spite of all you have endured, you appear to have developed a great sense of humour. There is often a twinkle in your eye when you mention the revenge that you would like to enact on Hets'. Annie chuckled and said that writing down her thoughts on paper had been quite helpful. It was the first time that she had done that. Annie had realized after the writing that she wasn't going to do any 'clobbering' but it felt good to vent her feelings, and she did want to become more assertive with people around her without going over the top. She had not sent her 'bill of divorcement' to Shirl but had decided to change her name by deed poll.

Annie then proceeded to tell me of a scene that she had dreamt twice the previous week. She was walking into a horseshoe-shaped building and saw a delivery boy spilling some cakes out of a tray. Annie went to help him and he gave her a piece of cake in appreciation. Annie's friends then came and took away the piece of cake. Annie said that she had been reading a book on Jungian dream interpretation to try and understand her dream. However, she said that she was sick of the author's style directing her how to interpret her dreams. 'The author says that each part of the dream has got to mean such and such', Annie growled, 'and I am pissed off at being told what to do!' 'Would you like to interpret your own dreams?', I asked. 'What do you think it all means?' Annie took a deep breath and said: 'Well, I never got any birthday cakes when I was a kid. I think the dream is about all the good times I missed out on and the cake I never had. And I think that all my straight friends are going to take any cakes that I might get now'.

We talked a bit about the new 'Rainbow Cafe' that had opened in Elwood and how gays and straight people seemed to mingle there, quite amicably, over the scrumptious food they served consistently. 'At any rate, since writing that letter I'm not going to let my anger at Hets win', Annie said. 'I'm going for a new job and I am not going to wear this T-shirt as I have done in the past'. As we completed the session, Annie winked and said: 'I'm into a real good book now. It's a sort of jokebook called *The Homicidal Lesbian Terrorist*.

I'll lend you a copy to read if you're not too frightened'. Annie shared the jokebook with me and, a few weeks later, offered me the following letter and plan of action:

On Friday, I was upset, but during that time some things came to light about my emotional life:

1) I realized that if I hang onto my anger/ sadness about my mother and so on, all that will happen is she will always have a hold on me. Also I won't resolve it that way even if I did make her aware of these emotions towards her.

2) Also revenge is out, not only for legal reasons, but also it won't change the problem. The need I have to punish her would be a waste of my life.

3) Also the need to sort things out, so we can get on together, has gone because of the attitudes that make us different.

4) Finally, I'm not as angry about what happened in the past but more angry about having a mother lost to me. So I'm really pissed off about not having a mother figure than the crap that has happened.

So now I've bitten the bullet and have decided on these aims and choices:

1) The past with her has no bearing on today or tomorrow.

2) She is no longer my mother in spirit.

3) That I will not have contact with her until I deem so and even then it will be my way.

4) She will not be called on to support me in any way ie, advice voices or housing.

5) I will not under any circumstances go to the suburb in which she lives until she has died.

6) I will not discuss mother or anything relative to her to anyone except professionals, especially comments about what she does, says, who she is.

I have realized that I don't need her anymore, that the gay world is my family in any respect I know I've got what it takes to succeed in this world.

And it's going to get better.

These are my winning attributes: good at socializing, making friends, in relationships, organizing things, speaking out thinking for myself, listening, work, planning, being reliable, changing, being and giving in most aspects.

These are the things I need for the next six months:

1) join two or more gay clubs.

2) see if I can start a business or do training.

3) manage my money better, pay debts over anything else.

4) lose weight.

5) stop smoking.

6) work out at the gym.

7) get out more

8) change my name.

9) stop being so reactive.

Discussion

The 'developmental, feminist and holistic maps' can be regarded as the contexts of the therapeutic conversation: considering the abuses and deprivation within her childhood that had laid the groundwork for her rage, examining the patriarchal thinking behind her stepfather's rapes of Shirl and Annie, and inviting Annie to step back out of her rage and start to look for the missing pieces that might lead to her healing. Some of the words that Annie used which enabled the therapist to imagine the real of her world were: fury raging within, wanting to clobber Fay, sick, hate, never praised, life a misery, laughed at. Whilst Annie certainly considered herself a victim of her mother's poor care during her childhood, she largely blamed the heterosexual world for the crimes which Shirl, her partners and her stepfather enacted against her (perpetrators of abuse can be regarded as viewing their victims within an I–It position). A story was used to encourage Annie to look at a different facet of the puzzle: that it was not the heterosexual world that was inherently conflictive but the irresponsibility of some heterosexual's perpetrators of abuse that gave rise to the struggles of the survivors. Telling Nasa's story can be considered an act of inclusion, joining Annie and Nasa as successful combatants against the harsher realities of life. Talking about the Rainbow Cafe can also be regarded as an act of inclusion, both gay and straight people socializing within an amicable environment. The contraries that can be considered reconciled were: Unconscious/conscious – using Annie's dreams as a resource to resolve her conscious emotional struggles; identity/identity diffusion – encouraging Annie to use her humour and creativity to develop her sense of self; homosexuality/heterosexuality – mentioning the good-willed interaction between customers at the Rainbow Cafe. Annie, in rehabilitating herself from drug and alcohol abuse, seeking therapy, changing her name and acknowledging appropriate attire for her job interview can be regarded as confirming herself as an effective survivor, rather than a victim, of abuse.

Case 3K: The mourning after

December, 1993: Colin, 18 years, an industrial engineering student, his sister Fran, 14, and their mother Valda, 51, a secretary, had all sought help together. Colin had tears in his eyes as he told me about his father's apparent lack of interest in him during access visits every second weekend. Nicholas, 48, a computer technologist, would promise to go camping or fishing with Colin, then cancel the arrangements because of work pressures. Colin would spend most of his access weekend watching television. Nicholas and Valda had divorced five years previously after a period of bitter verbal spats with each other. Nicholas had left to live with Simone, 32, a marine biologist. Colin admitted that the family atmosphere was much better since the separation, although Valda seemed to be still angry much of the time, screaming at Colin and Fran for no obvious reason. Fran commented that Nicholas paid much more attention towards her on access ('probably because I'm a girl and the youngest and Dad sees me as cute!'). She and Simone got on well together also. Fran felt that Valda 'dumped' her 'bad feelings' on Colin and her. Valda conceded that she yelled at the children a great deal, mainly because she could see how unhappy and angry Colin was and felt that it was all due to her fault as an inadequate mother who did not know what to do.

We discussed a number of themes that appeared relevant: Were Valda's feelings of being an inadequate mother due to community expectations that mothers have to handle any situation expertly, including their divorce and angry sons? In fact, I said I was admiring of Valda in her raising of Colin and Fran in the concerned manner with which they were discussing the family's struggles. I asked also if Valda was still mourning the loss of her marriage and displacing the anger of her grief onto her children? Was her anger a way of contacting the children? They were now growing into young adulthood; was there a more appropriate way of connecting with them so that they could all share their emotional struggles with each other? Would Valda start sharing some details of the family's finances with Colin so that he could help prepare a budget? Perhaps Valda, Colin and Fran needed to hold a Family Annual General Meeting to discuss their future direction? Would Colin let Nicholas know of some of the sadness that underlied his anger? Was Colin also grieving and was anger the only way permitted to men to express their grief within our society? I said that I valued Colin's trust of me in sharing his tears with me during this initial session and admired him for allowing himself to experience this soft side of his manhood. Would he invite Nicholas to a session of therapy 'without their womenfolk' to discuss some male stuff? Perhaps, underneath it all, Nicholas was grieving and his withdrawal from his son was a way of avoiding the pain of expressing his own sadness? As the family left, Valda sighed with relief, Colin offered me a warm handshake and Fran flashed me a bright smile.

Discussion

The 'developmental and feminist maps' can be regarded as the contexts of the therapeutic conversation: focusing on how the marital separation has come at a time when Colin is entering young adulthood and whether grieving in men is determined by fixed roles and behaviours. Some descriptions and behaviours which enabled the therapist to imagine the real of this family's world were: the tears in Colin's eyes; the parents' bitter verbal spats at the time of the divorce; the father's apparent lack of interest in Colin, his cancelled arrangements with Colin, and apparent favouring of Fran; the mother's dumping onto her children, her feelings of inadequacy and not knowing what to do. The contraries that can be considered to have been reconciled were: identity/ identity diffusion – Colin being invited to participate in a more adult role within the family – and intimacy/isolation – all members of the family being invited to connect more effectively with one another, within an I–Thou position. The Family Annual General Meeting can be considered an act of inclusion, inviting Valda, Colin and Fran to explore their future options together. The suggestion that Colin invite Nicholas to therapy can also be regarded as an act of inclusion, confirming Colin's ability to approach his father to discuss issues concerning manhood. Valda's self-recriminations as a parent are equated with the impossible community standards that are often expected of mothers (those people who label women as 'expert caretakers' can be regarded as viewing women within an I–It position) and she is confirmed as an effective caretaker, one whose children display sensitivity and respect towards their family.

Case 3L: Secrets revealed

November, 1993: Jane, 42 years, a journalist, came to her most recent session of weekly therapy in a flat panic. Having experienced several previous relationships with violent men, she had sought therapeutic help for about a year to explore different ways of relating to her partners. Jane had been involved for a couple of months in a friendship with Des, 38, a policeman, and she had been delighted with the respectful and sensitive way in which he had related towards her. That was until the last weekend. 'Des has just told me that he is a cross-dresser!', Jane exclaimed in anguish. 'He says that he wants to try on my clothes for size'. 'Hold on a moment', I responded, 'the fact that Des is talking to you about this matter indicates his sense of integrity. Have a sit-down with him and negotiate the rules'. Jane and I discussed what these might be: No cross-dressing in public; Des to buy his own clothes and not to wear Jane's garments; Des not to cross-dress when he and Jane are love-making. 'You may find that this is not the worst secret that a partner can reveal to you', I said. And how right I was!

Case 3L: (i) A dog's life

About a week after Jane had told me of Des's hobby, Gillian, 36 years, a cosmetician, and I met for the first time. She had been devastated by some news she had read about her ex-husband Max, 43, manager of a car rental firm. This couple had divorced two years previously after a seventeen year relationship that Gillian said had become 'stale and depleted', with hardly any affection, socializing or love-making between them. They did have one child, Patrick, now 17, to whom Max had proven a capable and committed father. Gillian had met Bert, 26, a gardener, soon after her separation with Max. Bert smoked marijuana regularly and was very much into 'male entitlements', dictating where and when Gillian was to work and seek leisure. Gillian said that her major problem with Bert was that he seemed very jealous of Patrick and demanded that she neglect her son's needs to tend to his own. Gillian had been struggling with whether to end the relationship with Bert or not when she had been flabbergasted six months ago to see a headline in the Melbourne magazine *Truthfully*: 'Man likes sex with dogs'. The article beneath the headline described how Max, over the past twenty years, had engaged in a '*ménage à trois*' with dogs and prostitutes and had taken photographs to be sold on the pornographic market. 'How could Max possibly prefer THAT to me?', asked Gillian in tears. 'Perhaps', I murmured gently, 'Max preferred sex with dogs because you weren't a bitch'. Gillian smiled, just a little. 'But I should have known that there was something going on!', Gillian continued. 'How could I have been so blind?'

I recalled the story of Kim Philby, the Soviet spy who lived with his English wife and children for decades in the United Kingdom whilst he conducted espionage against the British people. Suddenly, without a word of farewell or explanation, he disappeared, leaving his stunned family to grieve and wonder about it all. He surfaced many years later as a high-ranking KGB officer in Moscow. No one in his family had the slightest notion of his subterfuge whilst it was going on. I shared with both Jane and Gillian the following story from my own experience:

Case 3L: (ii) Unsighted

During the Family Therapy Conference in Brisbane in October 1991, I was chatting with Anne about the details of my *Family Counselling Casebook* which had been launched the previous evening. We had just met after attending the same conference presentation. I was standing in front of a long table, behind which Anne was seated and, as we talked, I flipped through some of the illustrations in my book. Although Anne was a lively conversationalist, I thought that she appeared a little bit vague in responding to the pictures that we were viewing together. After a couple of minutes, another colleague, Colin, came and whispered in my ear: 'You haven't sighted the dog yet, John'. I bent my knees, leant backwards, looked under the table, and came face-to-face with a beautiful Labrador guide dog. I gasped! Anne chuckled. My embarrassment was made a little less acute by the account of another colleague, Mark, who mentioned that he had seen Anne, during lunch-break, turning the pages and 'reading' the texts at the stall for newly available books. Mark had also thought that Anne was sighted until he saw the guide dog resting under the book display table and realized that Anne was getting 'a feel' of the books whilst she listened to the conversations of others around her about the various titles available.

This incident highlighted two points for me:

1. How my assumptions can be guided by my prejudices. I had not expected to encounter an unsighted therapist at the conference

2. How Anne's social skills had been so competent that both Mark and I had registered her initially as sighted.

Colin asked Anne: 'What would you have done if I had not alerted John to the situation?'. Anne replied: 'Oh, I would have let him go on until he found out for himself...they all do, sooner or later'.

We can all be regarded as making assumptions about the situations in which we find ourselves, based on the best information that we have at any given moment. I had assumed that I would meet no unsighted therapists at the Family Therapy Conference. Jane and Gillian had assumed that their partners would enter a relationship with them with honesty and trust. As it proved, Des was acting with some principle in telling Jane of his secret desires. When she negotiated some rules for his cross-dressing, the matter became a non-event and his yearning to wear female attire became much less. Their bond had deepened and they appeared more certain of each other. Max, however, continued to hide behind his sham, denying the verity of the magazine report and saying that he was framed by a fellow police officer who actually was the person involved. 'I thought you would have been the one person who would have believed me', Max accused Gillian, apparently trying to hook out her feelings of guilt. Gillian has gradually let her torment go over some weekly therapy sessions in which we discussed whether Max, Bert and Philby had all followed patriarchal scripts that allowed them to define their sense of masculinity to the disadvantage of their female partners.

Gillian is now working towards a separation from Bert and plans to start a new life for herself in England with her son. Patrick had gone there already to escape Bert's antagonism towards him and he had written to Gillian saying that he was looking forward to seeing her once more and to starting afresh, 'being a family again', amongst all their relatives who lived there.

Discussion

The 'holistic and feminist maps' can be considered the contexts of the therapeutic conversation: searching for pieces of the puzzle that underlie Jane's and Gillian's struggles. Some of the words that Jane and Gillian used that enabled me to imagine the real of their world were: panic, violent men, anguish, devastated, hardly any affection. I invited Jane and Gillian to imagine the real of my world: my embarrassment during the incident with Anne. Jane seemed to fear that Des's cross-dressing would lead to a life of deceit, but in fact he appeared to be opening up an avenue to discuss and resolve this issue. Max had kept his secret from Gillian who found out in the most painful way how she had been hoodwinked for so many years. When Gillian approached Max, he not only denied the story but blamed Gillian for doubting him, clearly indicating his guile in trying to manipulate her into a position of support for him. My story illustrated that a false assumption on my part influenced me to miss an important piece of information about Anne and that, conversely, what was not known led me into making an erroneous assumption. Anne appeared to accept my gaffe as an honest mistake. So, 'assumptions', 'secrets' and 'integrity' can be considered as pieces of the puzzle discovered. Max, Bert and Philby can be considered as lacking in integrity, all viewing their intimates within an I–It position and using them for their own purposes, whereas Des can be regarded as approaching Jane within an I–Thou position, willing to risk losing his relationship by revealing his secret openly to her. Rather than weakening their intimacy, through negotiation they both were able to enrich it. The contrary that can be considered reconciled here is intimacy/isolation: Jane and Des bridging the distance created between them through discussing their differences honestly and Gillian emotionally 'letting go' Max after realizing the extent of his fabrication. Sharing these stories can be regarded as acts of inclusion, connecting Jane, Gillian and myself within the communal network and confirming our humanness, as people trying to understand our assumptions about our world.

Case 3M: Intimidation

December, 1993: Simon, 20 years, unemployed, was telling me of his sense of disconnection with the outside world that had been present since his late primary school days. He had been very mistrusting of others since 13 years of age and, on occasions, had 'heard his friends voices in his head' speaking to him in his head since that time. However, Simon said that he definitely knew that these voices were psychological, in his mind, and not the influence of some outside force. Simon said that he was afraid of growing old, 'bitter and alone like Dad'. He described his father, Henry, as a cold, depressed, withdrawn man who had never been available to him or his brother, Ken, 23, for physical affection or conversation. Henry had finally hanged himself two years previously. Simon remembered his mother Winnie as a warm and generous caretaker during his childhood, always supportive and praising of her two sons. She had tried to excuse Henry's behaviour by saying that he had been emotionally abused by his own mother, particularly after Henry's father had been killed during the Second World War. Simon could not understand, therefore, why he was now struggling. Winnie had given both Ken and himself 'oodles of love' and every facility to succeed, and although Henry had 'not been there', he had never verbally or physically abused them. I asked Simon if he had been frightened of Henry and he replied: 'Oh sure. I'm not certain why but I was terrified of him. I think that Ken was frightened even more so; he will not visit Dad's grave'. Simon remembered that he and his brother had stopped talking to Henry when Simon was about eleven years old.

We talked about 'Mother's love'. It was expected to withstand all stresses and heal all wounds, yet often, when a father was an intimidating presence within a family, mother's love just wasn't enough to protect the children. Nor should it be! Children needed the care, sustenance and contribution from both parents, not just one. There also seemed to be a family tradition of emotional deprivation by the men within Simon's family. Henry, having been denied nurturing due to his own father's early death, perhaps did not know how to father his own children.

We talked about the 'seething rage that can underlie a cold exterior' and I said that Simon's account of Henry's manner had brought to my mind the image of a dormant volcano, ready to erupt at any moment. People who lived on the side of such a mountain could grow abundant crops from the rich black soil that lay on its slopes but they would live in constant anxiety of one day being swept away by a lava flow. Sometimes, withheld anger such as Henry's can intimidate children as much as a visible display of fury. At least with open rage, you know when to get out of the way, but with a dormant volcano, you never know when it is going to blow.

I shared with Simon a story from my own experience, one told to me by my mother Eva:

Case 3M: (i) Discipline

Eva was born in Upper Silesia, Germany, in the early months of World War One. Eva's mother, Marta, a schoolteacher, was a refined and cultured lady who had suffered many disappointments in her life. Marta's greatest sorrow was that she had wanted to marry a man of her own choosing but her family had decided to arrange a marriage to Ino, who was to be Eva's father. Marta seemed never to have forgiven both families for this forced match and she developed a smouldering hatred of Ino. From the beginning of war in August 1914, Marta was compelled to assist in the office of the family hardware store under the supervision of her mother-in-law, Rosalie. In mid-November, Marta was sent to Berlin once the advancing Russian Army's guns could be heard. When a retreat was established, Marta returned and gave birth to Eva one month early. Eva's misfortune was that she, an only child, resembled her father physically and Marta appeared to have displaced her anger for Ino onto her daughter. Eva's first four years of life appear to have been especially difficult. Ino was away serving in the Kaiser's army as a medical orderly on the Eastern Front. For much of that time Eva was deprived of emotional nurturing from either of her parents, being cared for more formally by Hedwig (or Hedla as Eva fondly called her), the general factotum and housekeeper originally employed in the home of Marta's parents. As Marta could not even boil an egg, her mother thought it wiser to install Hedla in Marta's new abode. When Marta did tend to Eva, it appeared to be in an abusive fashion. Marta did not violate Eva physically but rather in the form of very strict discipline.

When Eva was a toddler of about three, Ino brought home the Nagaika, a Cossack whip which a grateful POW patient had given him. Marta first threatened to use the Nagaika on Eva when she was a little over four years old. Eva had returned home from a friend's place later than permitted. Eva's little playmate, a lad who lived in the same building, had been doubly orphaned within the last few weeks. His father had been killed on the Western Front and his mother and baby brother had succumbed to the 'Grippe', the horrible influenza epidemic which killed more than the War. The boy's thoughtful grandmother had given her grandson a pair of bunnies and he and Eva had been engrossed in watching Mummy Rabbit give birth to her little ones, and so forgot all about the time.

Marta did not punish Eva immediately but waited until Ino came home on leave. Eva was called in solemnly after the main meal. Marta walked in carrying the Nagaika, told Ino of their daughter's misdemeanour and asked Ino to proceed with the punishment. This, of course, he refused to do, especially after so much time had lapsed since the 'crime' had been committed. Instead, Ino decided to give Eva a test and asked her to tell him what time the grandfather clock said. Eva smiled and answered correctly. Her little playmate was an 'expert' in not only telling time but also in taking watches and clocks to pieces and reassembling them faster than a child could say: Minute! Almost at once, Hedla returned to her original employment, before Marta dismissed her. After all, Hedla was (considered by Marta to be) a conspirator, being able to see Eva and her playmate, from the kitchen window, playing by the rabbit hutch. Eva was enrolled in the Jewish kindergarten, spent the afternoons with her cousins (Ino felt that the harmonious atmosphere of his sister's dwelling would be more suitable for his daughter) and walked home with her parents to sleep. Ino and Marta shifted into a new apartment and so Eva lost contact with her young pal.

Marta had always told Eva emphatically that her tenth birthday would be an extra special one, having gained double figures and started High School. Marta planned the biggest party ever for her daughter, with invitations sent out to twenty-five boys and girls. On the morning of such an event, the presents were usually displayed on a small folding side-table. The birthday person was led by their family into the dining-room ceremoniously, to the playing of a march and the singing of a tune. All this happened, but in the place where the presents were supposed to be lay the Nagaika! Ino, who was speechless, sent Eva out of the room and removed it immediately. He telephoned his sister and another aunt and asked them to take charge of the party, though Eva was only to learn of this later.

All that morning, Eva was as scared as could be. Came the afternoon, and the arrival of the guests, the procedure was repeated and, to Eva's surprise, in lieu of the Nagaika were flowers, a cake, books and, from Marta, an elegant box of printed greeting cards (which Ino and the aunts had overlooked). Within the box, each of the cards bore a different and viciously slanderous appellation, such as: Eva, the untidy one; Eva, the slow-coach; Eva, the lazy one; Eva, the peevish, grumpy one; Eva, the impolite, etc. When the aunts saw Eva's horror-struck face, they took the box out of her shaking fingers before the guests could see them. Eva refused to go near the Jewish print shop for months, for shame of what they might think. Ino's parents had given Eva a white roccoco-style writing-desk and chair and the aunts had added a desk-lamp and a rug. Ino, forgetting Marta, had suggested a proper wardrobe and this item of furniture became the bone of contention between Marta and Eva all through her adolescence. Needless to say, Eva learnt not to ask Marta for anything that she might have needed as she was growing into adulthood.

I asked Simon if part of his struggle was similar to that which my mother had experienced in her youth. Did he know how to ask for what he wanted? Perhaps the friends' voices that he heard in his head could be regarded as advisers, offering him wise counsel? Would Simon make a list of his needs now? At our next meeting, three weeks later, Simon showed me his list:

1/1/94 **My needs, qualities**

1) I need to know what is going on

2) feedback (does anybody like me)

3) a personality

4) a sense of humour (I want to find something funny one day)

5) I need to be able to talk, confidently and spontaneously

6) I need to be more than just a joke that nobody takes seriously

7) I need social skills and a satisfying social life

8) I need to have my own thoughts and opinions on things

9) I need to be capable of being liked by those whom I like

10) I need to be able to focus and concentrate

11) I need to be able to communicate

12) I need to break away from a) family b) others, *if* this is possible

13) I need to be able to explain *what cannot be explained* (so therefore my life is FUCKED and I wish I was dead, etc)

14) I need self-confidence

15) I need to be able to talk (to have something to say and to communicate it)

16) I need to be able to socialize

17) I need attention?

---

18) I need to be able to relax and trust others. I have none. I am a joke. If I have to I *will* kill myself; I suppose that is a strength. I think I have good intentions, but I can't communicate them (most of the time), so what is the point?

I cannot think of anything good about myself. I am a patheticuseless loner and I do not want to be like my father or brotherbut every day I can see something of my father in me. It is terrifying. I wish I was dead. I do not want to be this person for the next fifty years or so. Death is better. I do not want to be this person. I have a deep interest in spirituality, of whatever sort. I must not doubt this interest. I must know it is genuine. It does offer me some degree of hope (if I pursue it). I must pursue it, and from it I will gain strength.

I need to be able to cope with being on my own

I need dignity

I need to be able to assert myself

I need to be able to process and retain information in conversation, and when reading

I NEED CONNECTION'

Simon said that his mood had improved since compiling his list and I said how admiring I was at the clarity with which he *had* communicated his needs. Two major themes in Simon's list appeared to be: developing a sense of self and gaining strength from spirituality. Simon said that he often only 'felt who he was' when he was involved in an argument. I remarked that I believed therapy could help people to evolve both a sense of self and an intimate, spiritual connection with their therapist but that it might take a year or two of meeting weekly. Simon's interests were reading (period dramas like *Howard's End*; Simon was absorbed with the manner in which the characters related and 'belonged' to their family), films like *The Age of Innocence* (in which the characters tried to make some meaning out of the harshness of their situations) and music like that played by Madonna. I commented that I thought that if anyone could develop a sense of self out of chaos, it would be Madonna. Would Simon script a conversation with Madonna, seeking advice from her on how to mould personality out of confusion? Simon smiled and brightly bounced out of my room.

Discussion

The 'developmental, feminist, transgenerational, holistic and spiritual maps' can be regarded as the contexts of the therapeutic conversation. Simon wondered why his mother's love was not enough to have sustained him. Some of the words he used which enabled me to imagine the real of his world were: disconnection, mistrusting, terrified of cold, withdrawn, depressed father, generous, warm mother who gave her sons oodles of love. I invited Simon to imagine the real of Eva's world with the words that she had used in her story: scared as could be, horror-struck face, shaking fingers. We explored whether the community expectations of women as nurturers/caretakers was valid and whether, in fact, he needed both Henry and Winnie as caretakers working together to nourish him? Henry's emotional deprivation, due to his own father's demise in battle, and Henry's subsequent inability to nurture his sons was also explored. Henry appeared to have viewed both Simon and Ken within an I–It position, his sons being there to ignore. The description of Henry's withdrawal as 'frightening intimidation' can be regarded as the missing piece of the puzzle that Simon found. Telling Simon the story of Eva can be considered an act of inclusion: they are both survivors of emotional deprivation. In writing his list, Simon can be considered to be attempting to reconcile the contraries: identity/identity diffusion, intimacy/isolation and generativity/ stagnation and confirm himself as a person able to make his needs concrete. In contemplating a conversation with Madonna (i.e. an imagined dialogue with Madonna within an I–Thou position), Simon was invited to use his creative resources to experience both his sense of self and connection with the wider community.

Rather than write a conversation with Madonna, Simon chose to bring me a paragraph from Henry Handel Richardson's classic Australian novel *The Getting of Wisdom*:

> Of Pin she preferred not to think; nor could she dwell with equanimity on her late misfortunes at schools and the trials that awaited her on her reappearance; and since she *had* to think of something, she fell into the habit of making up might-have-been, of narrating to herself how things would have fallen out had her fictions been fact, her ascetic hero the impetuous lover she had made of him.
>
> In other words, lying prostrate on the sand, Laura went on with her story.

I asked Simon if he had given up on his life? If so, then his 'making up might-have-been' could be regarded as blaming the past for his current struggles. However, if Simon had not given up on his life, his 'narrating to himself how things would have fallen out had his fictions been fact', his 'going on with his story', could be considered a way of rehearsing for the future, exploring what optimism and hope lay in the direction ahead.

Case 3N: Cruelty

December, 1993: Robyn, 42 years, an unemployed stewardess, said that she had been 'unhappy' for the previous two years and was now feeling 'trapped' by the economics of her situation and the low income and poor job prospects due to the current recession. Robyn's life was filled with sad memories. Her father, Victor, an abuser of alcohol, had physically violated his daughter and her mother, Theresa, now 78, for most of Robyn's youth. However, Robyn's three brothers were treated like heroes and they also discounted their womenfolk. Theresa would not leave Victor for religious reasons and always made excuses for his violating behaviour. Robyn described Victor as a 'cruel bastard' who once found a litter of four kittens by the railway track and said: 'Look, magic! I can turn four into eight' and tore off their heads! Victor had died of emphysema ten years previously and Robyn had not visited his graveside since his funeral. Robyn had entered a four-year relationship with Ron, 30, a window cleaner, during which her son Graham, now 14, was born. Ron had shown no signs of commitment to the friendship. There had been little affection and Ron had left Robyn shortly after Graham's birth, without further contact. Robyn said that raising Graham, as his sole caretaker, had changed her life. She had learnt to develop love and trust with the other single parents that she had met on the way and, when Graham was eight, she met Peter, 40, an electrician. Peter had definite views favouring 'male rights' and 'men being the boss' but he did not physically or verbally abuse Robyn. The friendship had lasted six years and Peter and Graham appeared fond of one another. Robyn said that her main problem with Peter was that, whenever he took a stand, he was obstinate and would not budge. I expressed both my horror at Victor's sadistic behaviour towards Robyn and Theresa and my admiration that she had chosen to raise Graham and had gained so much from this experience. I asked Robyn if she would write a letter to Victor's 'ghost' contesting his abuse. Robyn wrote:

> To Victor Thomas Badman,
>
> I was a child – your child. I wanted to love you. I wanted you to love me. You didn't. I needed you to protect me and look after me as if I was worth something. You didn't. You told me I was worthless, no good – 'a thing!' Was there ever a time that you were glad of my

existence? My friend Nikki has a saying, 'Our parents don't teach us to be – they teach us how not to be'. You taught me how not to be.

I have a son named Graham. He changed a lot of things in my life. He taught me, without effort, what you couldn't. I delight in Graham and his ways. I hold him dear. I love him. I want no harm to come to him. I cannot envisage wanting to hurt him (or anyone else). I want the very best for him – not to punish, torment or destroy him. I wonder if you could understand.

It was my misfortune to have a father like you. It is the very best of fortune that I have a son like Graham. In reality one doesn't necessarily outweigh the other.

At 42, I now am faced with memories of you that I don't understand,with feelings out of control, with confusion. I don't want to feel sorry for myself more than I already have. I've always known you were bad, cruel, sick and vicious. It's just lately that I've realized the full extent of the misery you dealt out.

Over the years I wondered why you had such an evil nature. What made you like that? When I was small I used to think it was my fault. If I was really good and did everything to please you then you would love me – maybe even cuddle me – even a kind word. But of course that was the trick you played on me – just like the magic trick with the kittens. You had no love in your heart. You had no heart. I didn't understand. I was a small child.

When you were dying, even though I believe in fate, I felt sorry for you. It wasn't only because of your illness but because you could have had the love of your family around you. Instead we told real-life horror stories at your funeral. What a sad waste of a life!

Now that I am grown, I remember myself as that small child. I know the damage you have done. I know you to be evil and I hold you beneath contempt. If there is a heaven and a hell – then I know you are in hell.

Writing and sharing her letter with me seemed to have a liberating effect on Robyn. She had shared it with Graham who had given her a warm hug in return. During our next few weekly meetings we discussed ways that Robyn could assert herself more to Peter: Avoid 'Why?' questions and 'You' messages (Why haven't you changed the light-bulb yet? You said you would do it yesterday evening). 'Why?' questions often lead to blame of self and/or other (You are always nagging me to do everything. I can never get you to do anything promptly); Use 'Would' questions (Would you change the light-bulb tonight please?). 'Would' questions often lead to 'Which, How and What' answers which are usually not blaming and seek information (In which cupboard do we keep the light bulbs? How many do we have left? What strength do you prefer me to use?)

Discussion

The 'developmental and feminist maps' can be regarded as the contexts of the therapeutic conversation: examining how Victor's cruelty has affected Robyn during her growing years and exploring the patriarchal framework underlying Victor's abuse. Some of the words Robyn used which enabled me to imagine the real of her world were: unhappy, trapped, sad memories, father was a cruel bastard, little affection, learnt to trust and love through being Graham's caretaker. Victor and his sons appeared to have viewed all women within an I–It position: women had no inherent value of their own and were there to serve them. Writing her letter to Henry can be regarded as an act of inclusion, linking Robyn with all survivors who successfully contest their abusers. The contraries that Robyn can be regarded as reconciling in writing her letter to Victor, and examining the sort of questions she needed to ask to assert herself, were: generativity/stagnation, and ego-integrity despair. Our continued conversation invited Robyn to confirm herself as an assertive partner to Peter and enter into an I–Thou position with him.

Case 30: Comforting the crying child

October, 1993: Gabby, 36 years, an actor/singer and Hugo, 29, a secondary school drama teacher also interested in pursuing a vocation in acting/ singing, both attended our first meeting. They sat in my room with shoulders drooped, looking despondent and told me that they were low in energy. Gabby commenced to described her struggles. She felt that during the early stages of their seven-year friendship, Hugo had been preoccupied with his own needs and career development to the exclusion of her own. Although Hugo seemed to have improved in awareness and was more responsive to Gabby now, she said that she was brimming with resentment at his former apparent disacknowledgement of her. Hugo agreed with Gabby's assessment of the situation. He said that he had been self-focused and had discounted her requests but had become more aware of himself and had changed over the last couple of years. Hugo wanted to continue their relationship. Gabby related how life in her family of origin had been a strictly religious, joyless experience. She remembered it as always having been coerced to do 'the right thing' with little leeway for her own initiative or imagination. A family friend had sexually abused Gabby when she was eleven years old. Gabby's two younger sisters, and brother, were also troubled by depression and alcohol abuse.

Hugo described life in his family of origin as basically a happy one. 'Dad was a good bloke', he said, 'although he did not say much to any of us kids (Hugo had an elder sister and two younger brothers). I think that he was a bit disappointed that I did not study to become a true professional – a doctor or solicitor or something like that. Mum was always lovely – gentle and devoted to us all'.

I admired Gabby for having survived such a seemingly autocratic family, and the violations that had occurred, and commented that it sounded as if there was a 'young, hurting child–like Gabby' inside her adult body crying out to be comforted. I shared with her a portion of an article by Susan Rose:

> In order to survive the abuse, children may become detached and may sense that they are watching over the self who otherwise is not being rescued. In this sense, there may be a 'splitting' of personality whereby one symbolically becomes one's own guardian angel. But the guardian angel has no power to act, no particular magic to practice, other than that of escape and witness. Until the two selves are integrated, re-united, and the guardian angel is enabled to tell the story of the abuse as witnessed, the self cannot alter the meaning, and therefore, the consequences of the abuse. (1993, p.12)

Gabby had mentioned that she liked writing (Gabby had regularly kept a journal in a book that bore the slogan: 'She is a saucy girl; she is fifteen years old') and I asked her if the 'caring Gabby' inside her would compose a conversation with the 'crying Gabby' and offer her comfort and guidance. Gabby shared her composition with Hugo and me a week later:

> Dialogue between a young, unprotected seven-year-old Gabby and Gabby, now adult, caring and understanding.
>
> YOUNG GABBY: I'm frightened, they're staring at me.
>
> WISE GABBY: Who is staring at you?
>
> YOUNG GABBY: Men, boys, women – adults with their eyes and they're cold. They pretend to be warm but they don't care about me.
>
> WISE GABBY: What would you like them to do?
>
> YOUNG GABBY: I want them to take the shutters off their eyes and look at me properly.
>
> WISE GABBY: What is properly?
>
> YOUNG GABBY: With love and kindness and happiness.

WISE GABBY: You think that they're sad?

YOUNG GABBY: Yes and I want to cry.

WISE GABBY: You can cry.

YOUNG GABBY: It's hard.

WISE GABBY: Why?

YOUNG GABBY: Because they're looking at me and they won't understand.

WISE GABBY: You can cry whenever you want to.

YOUNG GABBY: Really?

WISE GABBY: Yes. You can save it up if you want to.

YOUNG GABBY: It doesn't mean there's something wrong with me?

WISE GABBY: Absolutely not. Crying is good for your soul. It's water for your soul.

YOUNG GABBY: Thank you.

WISE GABBY: Do you feel these sad people want something from you?

YOUNG GABBY: Yes.

WISE GABBY: What is that?

YOUNG GABBY: They want me to make them happy.

WISE GABBY: How could you do that?

YOUNG GABBY: Pretend to be happy. Smile. Look pretty. I'm very pretty but it makes me embarrassed. Like I've always got to look good and I'm tight. Very tight. But pretending to be happy. I feel trapped.

WISE GABBY: What would you like me to do?

YOUNG GABBY: I'd like you to tell them to all go away.

WISE GABBY: Everyone?

YOUNG GABBY: Yes. So I can be by myself and just hang around. No eyes looking at me.

WISE GABBY: I don't think I can do that.

YOUNG GABBY: Why not?

WISE GABBY: Because you can't control what other people do or what is around you.

YOUNG GABBY: So you're stuck?

WISE GABBY: No… Yes.

YOUNG GABBY: Tell me what to do.

WISE GABBY: *You* tell them to go away.

YOUNG GABBY: Is it safe?

WISE GABBY: What do you mean?

YOUNG GABBY: They might hurt me. Get angry.

WISE GABBY: I will be there. I will look after you.

YOUNG GABBY: How do I know if you will. Is there a guarantee?

WISE GABBY: I will be there. You are not alone. I will take care of you.

YOUNG GABBY: I want all you bloody people with your bloody eyes and hands and sticks and cars to just leave me alone. I don't want to see you staring at me. Go away and leave me alone. Stop staring at me making me sick and worried all the time. I want to put mud all over my dress and in my hair and take it all off, take off my clothes and run around the garden screaming and singing and dancing. And I don't want you around. I don't care if you think I'm crazy because maybe I am. If you still like me then maybe that's OKay. Just don't expect things of me.

WISE GABBY: What things?

YOUNG GABBY: To make the tea and sing pretty things.

WISE GABBY: There are some that are saying that's O.K. You can throw mud and they might even join you.

YOUNG GABBY: Really? That's amazing.

WISE GABBY: I will introduce you to them one day if you like.

YOUNG GABBY: I'm not sure. I'm feeling better now. I'd rather just play by myself.

Over the next three or four weekly sessions we considered Gabby's struggles within a feminist context; how pretty little girls were supposed to be good and well-behaved, 'sugar and spice and all things nice'; how women were expected to live within the mores of a patriarchal society. Were many of the expectations within Gabby's family of origin geared towards the advancement of men (autocratic religious families often are) leaving little time for leisure and fun? In her conversation, the 'crying Gabby' seems to be yearning for enjoyment of screaming and singing and dancing. Hugo may have also faced some patriarchal conflicts with his father in choosing drama teaching, acting and singing as occupations which were not considered 'manly enough'. I asked Gabby if she would continue to ask the 'wise Gabby' how she would guide the 'crying Gabby'. I felt it was important to keep checking the competence of our caretakers. I also asked Gabby to compare and contrast the negative qualities of the 'old Hugo' of earlier years and the 'new Hugo' of present times and monitor what changes had occurred. As Gabby had said that it was the negative qualities that had troubled her, it was important to ascertain how Hugo had improved. I also asked Hugo to compare and contrast the positive qualities between the 'old friendship' and the 'new friendship' so that they could both measure the triumphs that they had achieved together with the passage of time.

'Well', responded Hugo, 'there certainly has been less tension between us and more enjoyment'. Gabby agreed, with a grin, 'Yes, we have been lovers twice in the past twenty-four hours'. The two of them had participated in lovemaking every two or three months before this time, Gabby having been reluctant to invest in their relationship whilst their conflicts remained. I was thrilled. I told them that after our last couple of meetings, I had been left with golden feelings that had warmed me for much of the subsequent day. Gabby and Hugo both beamed.

Discussion

The 'developmental, transgenerational, feminist, communicational and holistic maps' can be considered the contexts of the therapeutic conversation. Some of the descriptions and behaviours that this couple used which enabled the therapist to imagine the real of their world were: shoulders drooped, looking despondent, low in energy; Gabby – brimming with resentment, strictly religious, joyless experience in family of origin; Hugo – self-focused, discounting, Dad was a good bloke but was disappointed in me. Gabby's caretakers appear to have viewed her within an I–It position, a patriarchal one which determined the roles of little girls: to be pretty, to make tea and sing pretty little songs. Hugo's father, also viewing his son within an I–It position, was disappointed that his son did not achieve patriarchal expectations and follow a 'manly' profession. Like father, like son! Hugo can be regarded as viewing Gabby within an I–It position, expecting Gabby initially to support him in his career to the exclusion of her own (Generally speaking, a patriarchal framework can be regarded as one in which people view each other within I–It positions, expecting themselves and others to follow rigid, robotic roles, to the benefit of men and the detriment of women). The 'patriarchal scripts' within both families of origin can be considered the missing pieces of the puzzle discovered, which enabled Gabby and Hugo to examine how their development had been influenced by those scripts. Gabby is invited to clarify the communication between her 'caring' self and her 'crying' self. In so doing, she can be regarded as confirming her abilities to ask for what she wants. The contraries that Gabby and Hugo can be regarded as reconciling were: identity/identity diffusion, intimacy/isolation, generativity/stagnation and ego-integrity/despair. Comparing and contrasting the various qualities of their former and current relationship can be considered acts of inclusion: Hugo and Gabby were invited to communicate to each other how they measured the progress of their friendship; indeed, I believe that one of the tasks of all intimate relationships can be regarded as how partners mark their progress over time.

Case 3P: Hatred

September, 1993: Hortensio, 46 years, trained as a broadcasting technical operator, came to therapy seething with anger. He told me how he had arrived in Australia twenty years earlier from Argentina. He had not been able to have his media qualifications recognized and had worked in various administrative positions, currently being employed as a secretary for a manufacturing company – a post he had held for the past five years. Soon after his immigration, Hortensio had met and married Tanya, a teacher, who also had decided to make a new life for herself in Melbourne. They had two children Phillip, now 17, and Billy, now 15. Hortensio had termed their marriage as 'a disaster from the start'.

'She is a materialistic, grasping and selfish woman, doctor', Hortensio said. 'I did not realize it at first, but she, being an Argentinean native, has a hatred of me and all those of European ancestry. She has married me, doctor, just to have her revenge on me, to take as much money from me as she can get'. The marriage had ended five years later. Tanya had moved inter-state, remarried, and appeared to have obstructed Hortensio's every move to have contact with his sons. Hortensio believed that Tanya had turned the lads against him. He said he had received a continual stream of solicitors' letters endeavouring to extract money from him and all his financial resources were spent long ago in trying to defend himself. Nonetheless, he had paid maintenance for his sons reliably and regularly. Hortensio was now constantly worried about what further catastrophe Tanya might call down upon him. He had lost all energy and enjoyment at work and did not see much of a future for himself.

It seemed apparent to me that Hortensio was paralyzed by his fury for his ex-wife and, perhaps, his unresolved grief since the end of their marriage. I invited Hortensio to write a letter to Tanya (though not to send it) expressing his feelings about the whole situation. Hortensio brought his letter with him to our next weekly meeting:

It may seem strange that I am writing to you now but I want to express in this letter how much I hate you. My hate comes from deep inside. It grows and matures more and more as time passes by. I hate you because you have no morals and for all the wrong you have done to me over the years of a humiliating relationship. my hate grows and grows but I do not do anything against you. I hate you but I have peace of mind. I hate you because hating you is the only right reserved for me.

I was naïve in the mid-70s when I took the risk of trusting so rapidly someone I did not know, someone I had just met, someone who pushed me wrongly to satisfy her mere personal gain. It was the wrong interpretation of a nice dream I once had. I thought we were compatible, but we weren't.

We were in similar situations and you took advantage of my trust in you, my work towards a common future, my friendship became a waste. I was to live with a stranger for almost five painful years. A jail in my own home.

I did not have a wife, I did not have a friend, I did not have a companion.

The product of my sole work for our future was all taken by you. You have given me nothing but misery and complications. You stole my money again and again, and you still take my money now.

You never worked for me, constantly cheating, stealing, abusing. The children we were supposed to share you also stole, you stole my rights and you stole the love the children had for me. The very little friendship left after the separation you also took away at the court session of 1982 in Canberra when you told the court so many lies in order to get more money and pay for your brand new car.

You knew how distressed I was after five years with you sucking my blood and ruining me and you took the children interstate. You made it extraordinarily harder. I had to put up with you for so long and still worked hard to pay you, solicitors and costs to see the children in Canberra until you took them to Brisbane. Your new marriage brought even more misery to my life when you started using your new husband, his money and his family against me. Later on (as all this had not been enough) you also turned the children against me in order to remove the love the children had towards me.

It is wrong. You are wrong.

I hate you. I hate having to write to you or have anything to do with you. I do not even see you as the mother of the children. You are nothing. You know that you are inferior, you have gone too far and you know that there are no more horizons for you. Everybody is sick of you and if you still manage to satisfy your ego it is because no one wants to argue with you or for fear you may hurt the children under your control. You are less than the living product of what comes out from the rear passage.

Why didn't I say all this to you before? – because of fear of more problems. But now it is different, I expect nothing from you, you can do nothing to me, do not even know where I am. You cannot 'defend' yourself with lies, and I wouldn't read anything from you anyway.

All your accusations against me now start bouncing back and turn against you. I hate you and when I feel better I forget you. Now, I have fewer work opportunities and get very little money. But I learned to find happiness in economical things. I have a simple lifestyle, although I am richer and feel more relaxed than when I let you be by my side.

I also learned to think of the children and love them without seeing them. I only regret they are with you too much and become like you.

What a bastard you are, I remember how bad I felt about you by the time of separation, despite the fact that I was giving you so much without asking for anything, and much more than you ever had in your life, you were still putting things of mine in plastic bags and hiding them in your wardrobe or under the bed. You thief. I rescued you from things you used to do before we got married, stealing from your employer or cheating at the supermarkets, swapping price tags of goods in order to pay less for what you wanted. Or your shoplifting practices on Friday nights.

Why did I ignore the important indications of what you were? Why didn't I think of you doing all that to me before? I do not remember one single genuine good time with you. There has not been a single occasion you approached me asking for something other than money. You knew all the tricks of a most dishonest person, I simply hate you.

You are nothing, I shall never forgive you for what you have done. I am gradually forgetting you, and soon I will forget you forever. I do not want to know about you. I do not want to write to you. I do not want to see you again. I do not love you anymore. Please stay away from me. We were strangers then, we are strangers now. If you love the children, let them go. Goodbye.

Hortensio said that writing this letter had released a great deal of energy. He had known how angry he had been towards Tanya but writing the letter had impressed on him just how far he was along the track of letting her go. He was now looking towards improving his own financial future. Over the next three months, Hortensio moved into a rented caravan. He has approached a solicitor to sell the flat in which he formerly lived – which he owns – pay off his debts, and reinvest most of the balance. With the remainder of the money, Hortensio plans to travel around Australia on holiday. He had always wanted to live like a gypsy for a while but had never been able to motivate himself to do so.

Discussion

The 'communicational and spiritual maps' can be regarded as the contexts of the therapeutic conversation. Some of the words that Hortensio used that enabled the therapist to imagine the real of his world were: disaster, materialistic, hatred, obstruction, a jail in my own home. Hortensio can be considered as viewing Tanya within an I–It position, blaming her for the cause of all his ills. In so doing, he can be regarded as viewing himself also within an I–It position: he was the defenceless victim of Tanya's wiles, isolated in his helplessness from the rest of the community (generally, persons who blame and view others within an I–It position can be considered as viewing themselves also within an I–It position). Writing his letter can be considered an act of inclusion: I believe that we all need to communicate the depths of our rage at times and protest against injustices, perceived or real. The contraries that Hortensio can be regarded to have reconciled were: intimacy/isolation, generativity/stagnation and ego-identity/despair. The letter can be seen as enabling Hortensio to let his feelings go and overcoming the emotional barrier that has prevented him from moving forward and connecting with others since his separation from Tanya. Hortensio then looked towards his own future, confirming his position as a capable participant within the wider community.

Case 3Q: Violation

December, 1993: During our first meeting, Yasmin, 24 years, a hairdresser, told of her difficulties in a recent relationship with Halil, 27, supervisor of a schools department. Yasmin had met Halil during a vacation he was taking in Melbourne. The attraction towards each other had been instant. However, when Yasmin travelled to Sydney a few months later to spend a week with Halil and his family, she found that he had been preoccupied with his work, making very little time to be with her and leaving it to his relatives to entertain her. Yasmin said that she had 'grown cold' towards Halil, broken off the friendship and flown home early. Yasmin was now wondering how she might achieve a more rewarding intimacy next time with someone who was prepared to be more available to her?

Yasmin related how her cousin Aliye's father, Yusuf, now 59, had sexually abused Aliye,[10] Yasmin, and several other female members of the family, when Yasmin was aged between eleven and twenty. Everyone in the family knew that Yusuf was 'fondling' the young women but they did not protest for fear of bringing shame to Yusuf's wife and children. I expressed my outrage that Yusuf had perpetrated his violations for such a lengthy period within the family without any reprimand and that the cousins had been denied protection by other family caretakers. Recently, Yusuf had been discovered violating two of his grand-nieces and, when the family did speak to him about it at last, he begged with tears not to go to the police and bring him into disgrace. I asked Yasmin if she would write a letter (though not necessarily send it) contesting Yusuf's abuse. Yasmin wrote:

To Yusuf Yasaf,

I am letting you know that what you did to me through my teenagehood was absolutely disgusting, disrespectful and scared the hell out of me. I didn't know that someone who is a so-called trusted family member would try and come on to me with force, knowing that I always used to try to get away and was scared of you. I suppose that is where you had the power, thinking I was too scared to say something, but I wasn't. All along my mother and at least five to six other girls that you abused knew, we used to talk about it and we all hated you for it.

All I wanted was for it to stop but no-one said anything because we were protecting your wife and children who you also treat with great disrespect.

Thank God you are now out of my life because I never, ever want to see your face around me again.

It's such a shame you had to get your cheap thrills on young girls and teenagers. You weren't man enough to try and make your own

---

10 Another story about Aliye is presented in Gunzburg 1993, pp.323–7.

marriage work but you do have a case history now of abusing women sexually, verbally and violently.

You are a sick man and don't think all the praying in the world will save you from yourself…you WOMEN ABUSER'

After composing her letter, Yasmin had compiled a list of questions concerning her current struggles and what she felt she needed to become a fulfilled person:

Questions:

1. Should I ring my uncle's wife?

2. How can I become a strong independent woman without scaring people away?

3. I get confused with how much housework I should do without being taken advantage of.

4. Why do I have to keep working to feel at peace? Why can't I just be?

5. I need to feel in control of myself.

6. I ignore my uncle as if he isn't there. Is that healthy?

7. Is it true that we usually cause certain experiences to take place by the way we think? Do certain thought patterns determine what good/bad things happen to us?

8. In therapy, do you deal with the 'inner child'? Do I not get close to other people because I am not close to my 'inner child'?

Things that I dislike about myself -

(a) not having the time/energy to talk to certain family members about how they feel.

(b) shutting my ear off to things that I don't want to hear.

(c) Feeling guilty about spending money.

(d) the shape of my body.

(e) afraid to take chances.

(f) I have no real close friends, too busy, get too cramped.

I congratulated Yasmin on both her letter and her list. I felt that she was aware of her dilemmas, had described them clearly and would certainly be able to resolve most of them during therapy. We discussed why men like Yusuf violate children and young women and the patriarchal attitudes that give them 'entitlements' to instant pleasure. Many survivors of abuse did struggle with developing intimacies within their communal network and I hoped that therapy would provide a safe haven, an oasis where Yasmin could come and refresh herself, tossing various ideas around and building up both her sense of self and a safe connection with me as her therapist. We concluded the session with a discussion of how, now that the family had confronted Yusuf about his abuses, Yasmin and her relatives could arrange 'safety meetings', ensuring that the more vulnerable family members were protected.

Discussion

The 'developmental, feminist and holistic maps' can be regarded as the contexts for the therapeutic conversation. Some of the words that Yasmin used that enabled the therapist to imagine the real of her situation were: instant attraction, grown cold, disgusting, disrespectful, scared. Yusuf's violations and their effects on Yasmin and other family members are explored. Yasmin labels Yusuf as 'sick' but therapy highlights another piece of the puzzle for Yasmin to consider: that Yusuf is following a patriarchal script, regarding his victims within an I–It position, to his benefit and the disadvantage of so many others. Yasmin describes her struggles in being able to feel good about herself and in enjoying social relationships. Violations can be considered as decreasing abused people's ability to form intimate I–Thou relationships. The contraries that Yasmin can be considered to be reconciling were: identity/identity diffusion, intimacy/isolation and genera-tivity/stagnation. Yasmin's letter and list can be regarded as confirming her ability to assert herself and ask that she be heard. The concept of 'safety meetings' can be considered an act of inclusion, inviting all family members to act in unison against any of Yusuf's future mistreatment.

Case 3R: An attempted reconciliation
June, 1991: Andrea, 34 years, an illustrator, and Richard, 32, a tiler, had separated four months previously after a four-year relationship. They had one son, Nigel, 2, and Andrea was telling me of her frustration at Richard's 'casual' attitude towards making any substantial contribution to family life. Richard smoked marijuana and regularly got drunk on weekends with his mates. He enjoyed playing with Nigel but rarely took any practical care of him. Richard worked part-time and appeared loath to build up his tiling

business to produce a viable and regular income. Moreover, he seemed to discount Andrea's efforts to publish her first children's book as a venture of no real value. To supplement the family's income, Andrea undertook child-minding. Recently, Richard had threatened Andrea, had pushed her across their bedroom and thrown Nigel onto their bed. It was these abuses that had prompted Andrea to demand that Richard leave.

We discussed Andrea's family of origin. Her father was an unrelenting patriarch who willed that he be obeyed and Andrea's mother rarely challenged him. She seemed to compensate for her husband's tyranny by dumping her bad feelings onto Andrea, screaming at her and hitting her. Andrea's brother, however, appeared to have escaped these beatings. I commented that women in this family appeared never to challenge the men no matter how unfair those men were and that perhaps Andrea had learnt not to confront Richard over his lack of input into the family. Andrea said that Richard wanted to reconcile but she wasn't sure which way to proceed. His violence had frightened her. I asked Andrea if she would invite Richard to a joint therapy session to discuss the situation.

At our next meeting, a week later, which Richard attended, he said that he was saddened at the split and appeared genuinely remorseful over his violations of Andrea and Nigel. I queried whether he would be prepared to attend Alcoholics Anonymous, but Richard denied that he had a drinking problem, saying that he and Andrea's difficulties were that they had to learn to communicate better. I asked them both if they would sit down together and negotiate a Contract of Reconciliation. This they did, and Andrea showed it to me at our next meeting a week later:

Attempted reconciliation agreement

We (Richard and Andrea) mutually agree that a six-week period of attempted reconciliation shall take place. The aims of this reconciliation period are –

1) To provide Nigel with a stable, comfortable environment in the home that has best been organized to meet his current needs.

2) For Richard and Andrea to live together for a period of time, maintaining some aspects of individual existence (i.e. separate rooms) whilst attempting to develop a mutually acceptable household routine, and according to each other the respect and courtesy normally expected of any two people sharing a household.

3) For Andrea in particular to rebuild some trust in Richard by him making concrete attempts to effect the promises he has made to deal with the problems associated with his drinking.

4) For Richard to save enough money to enable him to secure other accommodation at the end of the six-week period, if the reconciliation is not successful. This part of the agreement is undertaken because of the difficulties Andrea would have both financially and practically in securing suitable accommodation as a single parent with Nigel.

5) If during the six-week period an incident involving violent or threatening behaviour occurs (similar to that which precipitated the recent separation), Richard will undertake to leave immediately and seek other accommodation.

6) Andrea will not be willing to attempt another reconciliation if such an incident occurs and a permanent separation will take place. Andrea and Nigel will then reside at the current address with the guarantee of no further harassment. Richard will have access to Nigel on mutually agreed visits.

7) At the conclusion of the six-week period, if Richard and Andrea have agreed that they wish to continue living together, the points contained in this agreement concerning any outbreak of violent or threatening behaviour, will stand as a guideline for decisions *re* accommodation in the future.

Date –

Signatures –

During the six-week period, however, Richard slipped into his former drinking patterns and they decided to separate permanently, without any violence. I congratulated Andrea that she had demanded that Richard tend to her and Nigel's needs for safety and that they were able to negotiate a respectful parting. Andrea continued weekly therapy to work on her building up assertiveness skills and self-esteem. A year later, Richard contracted cancer. He underwent surgery and chemotherapy which achieved remission. He has reduced his alcohol intake and has been involved in Nigel's parenting responsibly and reliably.

Discussion

The 'transgenerational, feminist and communicational maps' can be regarded as the contexts of the therapeutic conversation. Some of the words which Andrea used that enabled me to imagine the real of her world were: frustrated, casual attitude, discounting, no real value, threatened, pushed, thrown, dumping, screaming, hitting. Andrea and I discussed the issue of 'male rights', how her father, brother and Richard appeared to have benefited from 'patriarchal privileges' and how the women in the family did not challenge them. The men can be considered to view Andrea and her mother within an I–It position, women being there to obey. Andrea's mother also can be regarded as viewing her daughter within an I–It position, Andrea was to be a receptacle for her mother's negative feelings. The contraries that Andrea can be considered to be reconciling were: identity/identity diffusion, intimacy/isolation and generativity/ stagnation. The Contract of Reconciliation can be considered an act of inclusion, uniting Richard and Andrea in their attempts to negotiate a co-operative relationship within an I–Thou position. It also confirmed Andrea as a person who was able to forward her needs and have them met.

Case 3S: Nourishment

February, 1991: Derek, 45 years, a marketing manager, and I were discussing his sense of emptiness and lack of motivation that had dogged him since his childhood. Derek described life within his family of origin as a mixture of experiences, sometimes aching with loneliness, sometimes bustling with activity. 'Dad was always aloof and unapproachable when he was at home', Derek said. 'I think he cared about us but most of the time he was away inter-state or overseas on business trips. Mum was always occupied with keeping the house tidy. She asked us to help her. We were a lively family, always doing things, but there never seemed to be much fun going around'. Nonetheless, the family did participate in many social and church-oriented activities when they were all together and Derek remembered the most enjoyable times as those when his parents had their friends over. Derek told how he constantly sought new challenges and ventures but rarely completed them. He had achieved a diploma in business management but had never stayed in one job for more than a couple of years. In fact, he really liked his current job of seven months and wanted to stick at it if he could.

Initially, I was not able to imagine the context of Derek's struggles. His parents did not appear to have been abusive or depriving and I wondered to myself if some event had intimidated Derek early on and that he had 'closed over' emotionally and not taken in many of the good experiences within his family that had subsequently occurred. Derek said that he could not remember any particularly nasty moments within his family as he was growing up. I commented that sometimes, for reasons not immediately clear, we experience difficulty 'belonging' to our families and that this leads to struggles in finding a 'place to belong' in other areas of our lives. Derek had said that he liked writing and gained much support from his Christian faith. I asked Derek if he would compose a list of some of the positive qualities that his parents had given him, qualities which now affirmed him and helped him to know who he was. At our next weekly session, Derek shared two lists with me:

Ways my mother and father created positive impact

1. By showing the importance of the domestic dwelling (home) as in shelter, food, ambiance, security, etc.

2. A realization that life has its many down times and the need to persevere along.

3. The importance of friends and spending time enjoying their company, i.e. a good sense of sociability.

4. That both, at times did express their love for me.

5. From my father, a sense of dress/style or better still a sense of stance or posture.

Ways that my mother warmed me

1. By praising my achievements and efforts. I spent vast amounts of my childhood doing housework, cleaning etc. I also got good examination results.

2. By showing affection and love physically – cuddling, hugging.

3. By responding to my storytelling and descriptions of my world and the events and things in it.

4. By humour, which is a shared reaction and children love to laugh.

Since compiling these lists, Derek described his mood as brighter, more alive, and we talked about how therapy could be rather like a treasure hunt, finding resources that we had thought were not there or that we had thought we had forgotten. I asked Derek that if he were truly contented, what would it feel like? Derek wrote:

If I were contented: more serene, calm, even-keeled, definitive, purposeful, rhythmic, as morning follows night, as the trees outside the kitchen window appear refreshed in the early morning wet, a more encompassing view, more balanced, less fear, worry, drugs, less fixation of self, more openness to people, a better sense of space.

We discussed the Biblical passage describing Moses' encounter with the burning bush and hearing God's voice declaring: I AM THAT I AM. I asked Derek who were the voices that had spoken to him when he was young? Derek wrote:

My guardian Angel – as conscience, mentor and advisor – was a constant voice in my very young years, providing a sense of balance to the various elements of life.

And I think that nature spoke (as it does to many) about beauty and the magnificent spectacle of life.

And so our weekly meetings continued for twelve months, emphasizing those parts of Derek's experience with which he could acknowledge himself as genuine and alive. I met him two years later, still working and enjoying the same managerial position.

Discussion

The 'developmental and spiritual maps' can be considered the contexts of the therapeutic conversation. Some of the words which Derek used that enabled the therapist to imagine the real of his world were: emptiness, lack of motivation, a mixture of experiences, aching with loneliness, bustling with activity, aloof, unapproachable, never much fun. As can happen, there is no obvious pattern within Derek's family of origin, no abuse or deprivation, to signal why Derek felt low in confidence and motivation. Perhaps he viewed his parents within an I–It position during his growing years: 'They should have been more loving, they should have done this or that, they should have been PERFECT parents'. The contraries that Derek can be considered as attempting to reconcile were: identity/identity diffusion, intimacy/isolation and generativity/stagnation. Whatever, Derek had not developed a firm sense of self and belonging and it was through writing his lists and descriptions which can be regarded as acts of inclusion, that he was able to confirm his sense of integrity and connection with others, including those people within his workplace.

Case 3T: Teasing

October, 1991: Cheryl, 17 years, a Victorian Certificate of Education student, told me of her anger at her father's discounting and teasing attitudes. 'He's always making fun of me', Cheryl complained, 'as though I will never do well'. Cheryl appeared to be experiencing similar patterns of behaviour within her intimate relationships. Her boyfriends mocked her also and she soon broke off the friendships with them. I asked Cheryl to write a description of the father whom she would have liked to have.

Cheryl wrote:

> Father,
>
> Kind, loving, willing to help, listen to problems, understanding, caring, gives good sound advice, gives hugs without being asked, doesn't feel funny about a kiss goodnight, smiles a lot, doesn't smoke or raise his voice like we are deaf.
>
> I don't care about how much money he has got. We can live in a caravan for all I care but I would like a father who opens his heart and discusses things without even asking you 'What is wrong?'; that would be nice.
>
> Somebody who would get my life in order.
>
> Somebody who would have taught me what organization is. Somebody who could have given me support.
>
> Somebody who doesn't expect too much.

After Cheryl had shared her description with me, we spent a few weekly meetings about how she might assert herself and ask her father to acknowledge some of her needs. To her surprise, after about six months, Cheryl said that her father had 'quietened down a lot' and was leaving her alone. She also had met 'a rather nice' boyfriend who did not seem to be 'giving her the jib' that so many others had done, and we concluded therapy.

Discussion

The 'developmental and communicational maps' can be regarded as the contexts of the therapeutic conversation. Some of the words which Cheryl used that enabled the therapist to imagine the real of her world were: my father's and boyfriends' discounting, teasing attitudes, always making fun of me, mocking. Cheryl's father appeared to have viewed her within an I–It position, Cheryl seemed to have been just a figure of his fun without any needs of her own. Writing her list can be considered an act of inclusion, inviting Cheryl to explore how she can join with others within intimacies and communicate her needs to others, asking to be heard. The contraries that Cheryl can be considered as reconciling were: identity/identity diffusion and intimacy/isolation. Successfully requesting that her father acknowledges her and that her partners treat her with respect can be considered as confirming Cheryl's abilities to participate mutually within relationships.

Case 3U: Immeasurable pain

July, 1992: Gina, 34 years, a receptionist, was devastated over the death of her husband, Tony, 36, an electrician, three months previously. She said that she had been talking to him on the telephone during lunch break, then, fifteen minutes later, she had 'felt his presence' come and give her a hug'. Gina said that she had intuitively known at that moment that Tony had died, and when the foreman knocked at the door forty-five minutes later, she had expected him to tell her that Tony had been killed, electrocuted at work. Gina was three months pregnant when Tony died. I asked Gina if she would put her feelings down on paper. Gina wrote:

> I miss my friend
>
> Ever since we have been together, I have had a fear of losing my beautiful Tony. Sometimes I would scare myself just thinking 'What if he left me?' or 'What if he died?' How would I ever live without him? So I'd think to myself that God would probably take me first anyway. I would push horrible thoughts of losing Tony out of my head, only to have them resurface again and again. He would always tell me to think positively, not to think of negative things and to enjoy myself instead of dwelling on depressing thoughts and working myself into a paranoid state. Our love was 'immeasurable', that's what we used to say. I'd say 'how much do you love me?' and Tony's reply would always be 'It's immeasurable' He loved to be cuddled. He was warm and giving as a best friend, lover and husband. He was sensitive and would shed a tear often at any sad happening in the world or to anyone near him. He would also shed a tear at the thought and or sight of a baby or child. he couldn't wait until the day that our own little one would be born. He worked hard, was honest, nobody didn't like him. I never heard a bad word about him. We would fight at times and they could be little spats to great big screaming matches. But we always kissed good-night and good-morning and never spent a night apart, except before our beautiful wedding day nearly eight years ago.

He made me feel so special and I was proud and extremely happy just like Tony when we found out six months ago that I was expecting our first baby. He couldn't keep it a secret, everyone knew. Tony had been working hard the last few months so when the baby came he could spend time bathing and cuddling and going for walks with the pram. We never took what we had for granted. Plenty of times we'd walk and say how lucky we were. There are others we know who mistreat their children, are unfaithful to each other, and are disrespectful of each other, but they go on unscathed.

Simple things like going to the supermarket together to shop at night or walking the dog on the beach occasionally; cuddled up watching television or sitting on the river bank when we got the chance. These things we always appreciated and enjoyed together. we didn't need fancy holidays or cars or restaurants. We just loved being funny and cute and then serious the next minute. Tony was my life. I only felt alive by his side. Why punish me and our baby? Why take away my beautiful Tony? I will never physically touch him again or his moustache or eyebrow or ear. He used to like that. I just cannot understand why he had to go now. Since that day the foreman came to our door, I don't feel alive. I feel numb and sad and devoid of any other feeling. I go to bed lonely and wake the same. I hear his voice all the time. I sleep on his side of the bed now. His photos are all around the house as they have always been. I can feel him with me and the baby. Any strength I have is only because of Tony. Is this God's test for me? Is this God's punishment for me? Was I so naughty once or twice or three times and over the years He saved up to get me this way? This is cruel. There will never and could ever be another like Tony.

With all my body, heart and soul I love him.

I cry, then laugh, then cry again, and I know all along that this terrible nightmare is too true for me to pretend he is walking back into our home. In the blink of an eye my life has been stripped bare. God, please don't let anything happen to our baby. That would be just the end. I will try my best for the baby but only for Tony and the baby's sake. I don't feel like I'm really here any more. I've been swept away in the rapids. Nothing stops, the world keeps going. Others have their tragedies too I know but my pain is my pain and I can't explain the depth because it is 'immeasurable'.

I shared with Gina a poem that a mother, dying of cancer, had written for her children:

When I must leave you[11]
When I must leave you for a little while,
Please do not grieve and shed wild tears
And hug your sorrow to you through the years,
But start out bravely with a gallant smile
And for my sake and in my name
Feed not your loneliness on empty days.
Beautify each waking hour in useful ways,
Reach out your hand in comfort and in cheer
And I in turn will comfort you and hold you near
And never, never be afraid to die
For I am waiting for you in the sky.
I love you all, just remember that.
Faith is like a shining star
Beckoning us from afar.

Sharing these pieces of literature appeared to offer Gina some relief. Over a series of weekly sessions, she gradually let the pain within her grief go and looked more towards the future after the birth of her and Tony's child.

Discussion

The 'spiritual map' can be considered the context for the therapeutic conversation. Some of the words which Gina used that enabled me to imagine the real of her world were: devastated, horrible thoughts, punishment, don't feel alive, cruel, terrible nightmare. Whenever tragedy hits us, it can feel like an isolating experience, as if the world, God, Nature is viewing us within an I–It position, cruelly and heartlessly. It is at these times that sharing literature within an I–Thou position can be an act of inclusion, connecting us with the experiences of others who grieve. We can join with those others, find our comfort and, in doing so, can be regarded as reconciling the contraries generativity/stagnation and ego-integrity/despair.

Case 3V: A different angle[12]

May, 1992: Mary, 35 years, had brought her son, Patrick, 7, to therapy because of his quiet, sad demeanour that had developed over the past few weeks. Previously a happy little lad, Patrick had become reclusive, staying

---

11 This poem was originally presented in Gunzburg 1991, p.113.
12 This case was originally presented in Gunzburg 1994.

in his room for hours after school and missing his favourite television programmes. He had ignored the invitations of his many friends to come over to their homes and play and his school teachers had noted Patrick's decreased participation in class activities. During our conversation, Mary mentioned that her father, Damon, 75, had died three months before after a short battle with cancer. Mary thought that Patrick missed his 'Grandpa' enormously and she expressed her own distress at her father's death, and at her seeming inability to 'cheer Patrick up'. 'Where do you think Grandpa is?', I asked Patrick. 'In Heaven', he responded solemnly. 'And what do you miss most about Grandpa?', I continued. 'Oh, he was great!', Patrick replied. 'He would take me to the park to play and buy me jelly beans, those really yummy purple ones'. I asked Mary if there was anyone else who might take Patrick to the park occasionally and buy him those very special sweets, as Damon had done. I also asked Patrick if he would draw a picture of Grandpa in Heaven.

At our subsequent, and final, session three weeks later, Mary related that both she and Patrick were much easier in themselves and that Patrick had resumed his usual routines. An uncle had taken him twice to the park and had bought him 'Grandpa's treat'. Patrick showed me his picture of Grandpa in his new Heavenly home, smiling, and playing with many angelic friends that he had made there. Patrick had entitled his drawing: *Grandpa in Heaven, with all the Angles.*

Discussion

The 'spiritual map' can be considered the context of the therapeutic conversation. Some of the words and actions which this family used that enabled the therapist to imagine the real of their world were: quiet, sad, reclusive, Patrick ignoring invitations of his friends to play, his decreased participation at school, Mary's distress. Mary berated herself that she was unable to help Patrick regain his equanimity. She can be regarded as viewing herself within an I–It position: that she needed to be a perfect mother in every situation. Mary was invited to reflect that Patrick's sadness was a very ordinary response to Damon's passing. A relative was found to continue some of the pleasures that Patrick had enjoyed with his Grandpa and Patrick expressed some of his grief through artistry. The contraries that can be considered to have been reconciled were: intimacy/isolation and generativity/stagnation. Both of these events can be considered acts of inclusion, connecting Patrick to others within his family and to the spiritual world.

Case 3W: No obvious losses![13]

August 1992: Leo, 37 years, and Coral, 33, and their three children, Max, 6, Tina, 4, and David, 2, had sought therapy because of a number of problems. Coral described her constant tiredness. Leo worked long hours at the television studio as floor manager, and this included most weekends also. Coral was left to cope with the children. Tina had begun soiling her underwear six months previously. About the same time, Max had taken to throwing tantrums and messing the house with his toys, dirty dishes and food scraps. On drawing the family's genogram, there were no obvious losses and I anticipated that we would meet every 2–3 weeks, during which we might weave some themes around marital and parental issues, help Max to 'tame his temper' and, for the moment, take the focus off Tina's soiling. Max said that he missed his Dad and we talked about how Leo might spend an hour's 'caring time' with Max and Tina, giving them some of the company that they might be wanting. I asked Max if he would draw a picture of his temper for a subsequent session, with the eventual aim of putting it in a 'temper box' and, with the encouragement of other family members, helping him to contain it in there.

I introduced the theme of 'parental expectations' into the conversation: how parents, in traditional families, are expected to be super-effective – mothers taking on the burden of domestic chores, whilst fathers go out bravely to support the family by earning income. I affirmed Leo and Coral as dedicated parents, obviously concerned for their children, and wondered if all their energy was going into parenting and little into marital fun. We discussed ways that Leo and Coral might make their relationship 'special': watching a video together, a night out for pizza and coffee, a walk in the park. I also wondered if Max was learning from Leo that certain chores are 'women's work' and that he was leaving his rubbish around for his mother to pick up. We organized a Gold Star Chart: if Max could keep the dining-room, lounge and hallways clean of his rubbish five days each week, he would be awarded a silver star. If he could keep those areas tidy three weeks each month, he would get a gold star. Two months and two gold stars in a row would lead to a special treat.

A few months passed and nothing changed. Then, as luck would have it, Leo developed gallbladder disease, required surgery and was off work for several weeks. During his rehabilitation, Leo looked after the children competently, spent time with both Max and Tina and prepared meals and participated in the housework in a way that Coral felt appreciated and rested.

---

13 This case was first presented in Gunzburg 1994.

Tina's soiling and Max's tantrums and sloppiness in public areas of the house had ceased and I thought that I had achieved some fine results with structural, behavioural and a touch of pro-feminist therapy. I asked the family what they thought had caused the changes. 'Oh, it was when we got the new cat', Coral replied. 'Our last puss died a year ago (about the time Tina and Max started 'messing' around). It all got better when Tompkins came to live with us several weeks ago.'

Discussion

The 'structural and feminist maps' can be considered the contexts of the therapeutic conversation. Some of the words and actions which this family used that enabled the therapist to imagine the real of their world were: Coral's constant tiredness, Leo's long working hours, Tina's soiling, Max's outburts of anger and making a mess. Leo and Coral brought to therapy a number of stressful experiences in their family life: Max's tantrums and untidiness, Tina's soiling, Leo's long work hours, Coral's dissatisfaction. Perhaps Leo and Max were viewing Coral within an I–It position, that she be the exceptional wife and mother? A variety of themes were discussed: affirming parenting, increasing marital enjoyment, examining gender roles and augmenting Max's responsibility. The 'Gold Star Chart' and Leo's illness can be regarded as acts of inclusion, all members of the family joining around them. The contraries that members of this family can be considered to be reconciling were: identity/identity diffusion and intimacy/isolation. Coral signaled that re-placement of the deceased family cat had been a marked effector of change. This case, like (Case 3L (ii): Unsighted, p.150), proved yet another illustration for me not to assume that, at any given moment, I had all the information at hand during the therapeutic meeting.

Case 3X: Needs and wants

March, 1993: Steven, 42 years, a mildly obese nursing attendant, was describing his confusion, disorientation and lack of meaning in life. Four years previously, he had divorced Lydia, 42, dance teacher and wife of thirteen years. It had been an amicable separation and they still paired up for, and sometimes won, ballroom dancing competitions. There were no children. One of the reasons for the separation was Steven's strong sexual desire for other men, which had been present since his adolescence. Steven had currently enjoyed a friendship with Jack, 49, a builder, for the past eleven months but Jack appeared hesitant to make a commitment to a long-lasting partnership. Steven was also unsure. He warmed towards women emotionally, felt very comfortable socializing with them, but experienced no erotic desire for them. At age twenty-three, Steven had suffered severe panic attacks, thought that he had been going mad and had been certified and institution-alized for several weeks. He had been free of medication now for many years. Steven had decided to seek therapeutic help to ascertain whether he might try once more to establish a 'normal' marriage.

Over several weekly sessions, we discussed Steven's likes (ballroom dancing, Chinese food, musical theatre) and dislikes (social gatherings, travelling). He certainly seemed to be bi-sexual – loving conversation, hugs and massage with women but being 'turned on' by the visually-stimulating images of men. A crisis eventuated when Steven chose to holiday for two weeks in the Pacific Isles. He had been conned by a group of locals who had encouraged him to pay several hundred dollars to share their hospitality and join them in a feast. When reporting the incidence to the authorities, Steven was told to drop the charges or else face a significant prison sentence for being homosexual and corrupting the indigenous population.

Three months after therapy had commenced, Steven had lost weight and had entered an intimacy with Harold, 55, a storeman. They had moved into joint residence, a situation that Steven would never have contemplated before. I was admiringly amazed, congratulated Steven and asked him what had made the change. 'It was when we started discussing likes and dislikes some time ago', Steven replied. 'I came to realize that there was a difference between my needs and wants. What I wanted was a lifestyle that I perceived to be normal. What I need is a good-willed and 'whole' relationship with a person like Harold to help share the stresses I face whenever I socialize and travel'.

Steven decided that he NEEDED no further therapy!

Discussion

The 'holistic map' can be regarded as the context of the therapeutic conversation. Some of the words which Steven used that enabled the therapist to imagine the real of his world were: confusion, disorientation, lack of meaning in life. Steven appeared to have been viewed within an I–It position by many within the community who are prejudiced against homo-sexuality. I can be considered to be inviting Steven to join me within a respectful I–Thou conversation that acknowledges his right to choose his life-style. The contraries that Steven can be regarded as reconciling were: identity/identity diffusion and intimacy/isolation. The difference between what he 'needed' and what he 'wanted' can be considered the piece of the puzzle that Steven discovered to resolve his dilemma.

Case 3Y: A friend indeed!

April, 1981: Harriet, 48 years, a housewife, had visited my general practitioner's surgery to seek advice regarding a sore throat and, in passing, mentioned that her son, William, 14, had been apprehended the previous week for stealing. Harriet was smiling as she told me this news and, suspecting that there was a story to be told, I asked her how it had all come about.

Harriet replied that William was friendly with Brendan, 14, the lad across the road. Some weeks before, Brendan's father, Tom, had deserted the family without providing any financial maintenance or emotional support for his wife and four children. Brendan's mother, Frances, had become severely depressed and was coping not at all. The state of their house was deteriorating and Brendan and his siblings were being poorly fed and clothed. William had decided to take Brendan to the local supermarket and had shoplifted some food items. On catching the two boys in their thieving, the supermarket manager had contacted the police. Two police officers had approached Harriet the same day and had informed her that there would be no charge against either lad. Rather, the council social workers had been notified and proper care had been commenced for Brendan's family.

I told Harriet that I was impressed; William appeared to have learnt early that sometimes, in our society, the only way to obtain adequate help for a friend is to break the law!

Discussion

The 'holistic map' can be considered the context of the therapeutic conversation. Harriet's smiling as she told me that her son William had been apprehended for stealing made it difficult for me to imagine the real of her world until she had told me her story. William appeared to be a lad gifted in I–Thou relating. He seemed readily able to imagine the real of Brendan's situation. Recognizing that William's and Brendan's 'breaking the law' was an effort by one friend to help another in trouble, rather than the commencement of a criminal career, can be considered the piece of the puzzle discovered that gave meaning to the boy's actions. William's stealing can be considered an act of inclusion, inviting the police, the welfare workers, Harriet and me into the world of Brendan's distressed family. William can be considered to have helped Brendan reconcile the contraries identity/identity diffusion and intimacy/isolation and, in so doing, to have confirmed himself as a loyal mate.

Case 3Z: Tales my parents told me

The film *Shadowlands*, with Anthony Hopkins and Debra Winger, is based on the friendship between the English author C.S. Lewis and the American poet Joy Gresham. There is a beautiful line that Hopkins, playing the role of Lewis, speaks: 'We read to know that we are not alone'. I think that this is also an accurate reflection about therapy: we invite each other into genuine dialogue to know that we are not alone.

We also can tell stories to each other during the therapeutic conversation to know that we are not alone. The readers of this book will have realized long before now that I enjoy sharing tales and anecdotes. Actually, what I most enjoy is the interweaving of themes, the play of ideas and emotions, that occurs within the telling. If I could invent a name that would adequately describe my work as a therapist, it would be that of a 'theme weaver'. My aim is to invite readers to engage with the material, to participate within the stories, to experience the complexities of the people involved and their struggles, to engage with those struggles and not to back away from the ethical dilemmas faced, no matter how confronting they be.

I value also how stories connect us from generation to generation and from culture to culture. I appreciate how the stories include us all within their telling. The clients whose stories have been told so far privileged me with their knowledge and wisdom and were not withholding to have their stories re-told on these pages. They permitted me to share their journeys with them and to learn about a rich, sometimes painful, always inspiring experience on the way. So, I would like to conclude this section with two accounts from two of the most fulfilling story-tellers that I know: my parents, Noah and Eva Gunzburg. My parents and I have been blessed in sharing our journey for over half a century and I would like to invite readers into a world which my parents know (and with which Buber was familiar), a world gone long ago but which retains its flavour through their telling. Come and join us:

Case 3Z: (i) Grief resolved

My father speaks of his ancestors with quiet pride... 'The famous Baron Gunzburg, who lived in St. Petersburg in the late 1800s, was well respected and highly known for his work as a spokesman for the Jewish community. He was a friend of Czar Nicholas II and was able to prevent some of the antisemitic mischief of Rasputin. Baron Gunzburg died in 1909. Further to the East, in the town of Minsk, there were other branches of the Gunzburgs, and it was from these that we were directly descended. They were wealthy textile merchants and my great-grandfather Noah, after whom I am named, obtained a rare privilege in the form of a visa to live in Moscow. Some of our family had enough money to gravitate towards the Promised Land. My grandfather, Mordechai Freiman, was one of the founders of Rishon le Zion, Israel's first Jewish settlement in modern times, and another relative, Israel Belkind, founded Youth Aliyah, an organization that encouraged immigration of the young to Israel. His son, Naaman Belkind, spied for England against the Turks during the First World War and was caught and hanged. Another cousin, Avshalom Fineberg, was also an undercover agent for the British in the Middle East during the same period. Both he and Naaman were members of the espionage group 'Nili'. Avshalom was captured by the enemy, shot by firing squad and buried in an unmarked grave near Beersheba. Some decades later, a desert traveller resting by a young palm tree noted a white object protruding from the earth at the base of the palm. He dug a little deeper and uncovered some bones and a wallet identifying them as the remains of Avshalom Fineberg. Avshalom had been buried with some date pips in his trouser pocket and one had germinated to give rise to the palm. Avshalom's grave-site was now known and the grief of surviving family members could also be laid to rest'.

Case 3Z: (ii) The awesome days of Tishri

(My mother tells of her childhood memories of Beuthen, Germany, in the 1920s). 'These actually commenced for us on the last Sunday in Ellul prior to Jewish New Year, when we all picked up my grandparents to take them to the respective cemeteries to pay their respects to their forebears. First was the 'Old One', which was only opened once a year for that purpose. Towering wild chestnut trees threw shadows over the stones, some dating back to the 13th Century. Here was the stone for my great-grandmother, after whom I was called Chava. After lunch, we travelled into Poland to a small village called Nicolai, where my ancestors had been farmers and cattle dealers since the 14th century. The barn and old farmhouse still stood and there were rows after rows of ancestral graves. It was a lesson in history and genealogy.

On the evening of Jewish New Year, all Jewish premises closed early – be they Orthodox- or Conservative-owned. (The non-Jewish employees expected the two days off, as well as the Day of Atonement). Beautiful smells exuded from the kitchens whilst we dressed in our finery. Wearing our new clothes, my father in top hat and all of us with white gloves, we made our way to Synagogue Square, on the way meeting more and more congregants. The lights of the Synagogue shone out. As we entered, men and women left their overcoats, top hats, shoes and umbrellas in the cloakrooms in their respective foyers. There were three galleries for the ladies and children and seats for six to eight hundred men and boys. The choir loft held at least forty to fifty choristers. The pulpit, and ark in which the Torah scrolls rested, were clad in beautiful white velvet-embroidered cloth. There were seats for the Rabbi, Reader, Cantor, Usher, President, Vice-President and Treasurer, as well as several Ushers allotted to each section. As soon as you entered through the doors from the foyers, SILENCE reigned.

We proceeded quietly and quickly to our allotted seats and whispered to our neighbours: 'L'Shana Tova – A Happy New Year'. At the proper time, the doors of the vestry opened, the congregation stood respectfully and the dignitaries' boxes were filled with the aforementioned people. Last to enter was the majestic figure of the Rabbi. The Cantor and Rabbi, to the tune of Baruch Haba (Blessed be those who come), proceeded down the steps and walked in procession to the entry doors to welcome the mourners and guide them to their new seats (a mourner changed his seat for the year of mourning). Then the service began. We spread our white handkerchiefs and sat on the steps. The solemnity of the service was most impressive. The foyer doors remained locked during the reciting of Amidah, the Reading of the Torah and the Sermon.

At the end of the evening service we kissed and hugged our mothers, grandmothers, aunts, friends and teachers and made an orderly exit to the foyers to retrieve our garments. We were very careful to utter the appropriate address of 'L'Shana Tova Tikatevi' to the females, or 'L'Shana Tova Tikatevu' to fathers, uncles, grandfathers, brothers or cousins, as we had learned at Hebrew School. Synagogue Square was packed with friends and family and we slowly made our way back home to start the festive meal with all the traditional dishes: the round bread loaves, the apple dipped in honey, etc, etc.

After the service on the first day of Jewish New Year it was our custom to visit relatives on our way home, not immediate members like aunts and uncles and cousins but second cousins or more remote relatives whom we had not regularly visited during the year. A very warm welcome awaited us and there was a distinct order of whose house was called on first. The second day was similar to the first except that, after Synagogue, visiting was to close family friends.

During Jewish New Year, as well as the full 'Ten Days', we did not listen to the radio, play a gramophone, go to a cinema, theatre or other place of amusement. We even cancelled our music lessons.

Then came the Day of Atonement. We all made our way quickly to the Synagogue and it was a strange and solemn feeling to enter the main building. By the appropriate time, all seats on the men's level were occupied and extra benches had been added for guests and strangers. The first, and most of the second, gallery for ladies was packed out. Only on the third gallery were there a few empty seats. The cantor intoned the Kol Nidrei and the service began. We followed this part of the service from our mother's or father's Festival prayerbook as it was not in our regular prayerbook. The solemnity of the occasion seemed to pervade us all.

The next morning, my father left early to be at the Synagogue for the start of Morning Service whilst my mother and I usually arrived well in time for Shema and the morning Amidah. We children tried to follow the service from our regular prayerbooks. We only received a set of Festival prayerbooks for our Bar Mitzvah, or for girls, at age twelve. During the Memorial Service only orphans were allowed to remain inside. As this service usually lasted one-and-a-half to two hours, we left for the City Park. Incidentally, both my parents left too as my grandparents were all alive until the early 1930s. They just went to my aunt's place. In the City Park, we youngsters began the job of eagerly gathering up the shiny brown wild chestnuts to make chains for the decoration of the Communal Tabernacle. We returned near to Synagogue Square and emptied our pockets into a tub at the back of the Jewish fishmonger's shop where the tabernacle was awaiting erection.

We then proceeded quickly to the Synagogue to hear the Sermon and Additional Service. There was another short break before the Afternoon Service which we used to dash home (none of us lived more than ten minutes walk from the Synagogue). We returned to the Ladies' Galleries with apples or oranges, which were pierced with cloves to give a pleasant odour, to revive the flagging spirits of the mothers, grandmothers and aunts. The rays of the setting sun shone through the windows as the Closing Service was chanted. The beautiful melodies of Lewandowski throughout the Additional and Closing Services are still ringing in my ears. At the last Shofar call, we greeted each other with: 'Hope you have been inscribed in the Book of Life'.

A personal reflection

My father, Noah Gunzburg, writes of Mordechai Freiman and Rishon le Zion:

Once more the urge has taken seized me to burst into some mild but quite interesting prose on the days when I had finished primary school and, in 1922, sailed to the land of Israel with all the family.

The purpose of this was simply that in those days Jews were marrying out of their religion and this was a situation that my parents, in the love of their culture, wanted to avoid for us.

So off we went and what an experience it turned out to be. Rishon le Zion was founded by my grandfather, Mordechai Freiman. He had a lovely home and was the honorary magistrate for the local government. He was a very amiable and intelligent gentleman who spoke several languages. Among his guests was a Lutheran parson who wanted to convert grandfather to Christianity for, as the parson told it, how could a Jew speak such beautiful German? Just a few metres down the road was a beautiful synagogue which the town had built in grandfather's name, and he founded a string of Talmud Torahs in Rishon.

And now I want to touch on another scenario which goes right to my own heart. Remember, this was in the early 1920's, and the township of Rishon le Zion was still fighting hard to establish itself. Nevertheless, it had achieved a lot in agriculture, particularly in wine-growing. Baron Edmond de Rothschild had built his famous wine cellars and they were already fully working. The wine harvest, known in Hebrew as 'Hakatzir', was quite an event. It used to happen just at Pesach time. Let me describe to you one season I happened to witness in 1924. Outside the doors of the cellars was a huge tent with hundreds of guests sampling the wines. Next to the tent was an enormous weigh-bridge, and we would see the vignerons continuously driving their heavily-laden carts onto the weigh-bridge and straight to giant machines which immediately swallowed the whole cartload and transferred the juice into huge vats within the cellars. It was really a very stirring experience.

The spectacle could also be quite funny. When buying wine, our family used to go there to get all our Pesach requirements. The colonists, however, expected special privileges and sometimes there could be trouble with the very old settlers. They were used to the cheapest prices and would bring their own bottles along to get them filled. The cellars were against this practice as, under the direction of the Chief Rabbi, all the bottles are washed in water for twenty-four hours before filling them, to make them fit for Passover. So the cellars objected to the settlers bringing their own bottles. I never heard how that ended.

Somewhere in the offices of the cellars, there is a Daguerreotype picture of two little scamps with a long branch between them on which is hung a giant bunch of grapes. They look very comical as they carry their load, my Aunt Hassiah standing in the back, and my Uncle Harry in the front. The message is very clear they are enacting the story of Joshua's two spies. (Apparently, it was from this picture that Baron de Rothschild's 'Carmel' wines took their logo).

When you think of it, does it not give us much to be proud of this relatively small number of Jews achieving so much to the establishment of a township, and religion nonetheless not being neglected.

Epilogue

'My second story,' said Jaacob Yitzchak, 'is even briefer and more concise than the first. It's title is: "How I Apprenticed Myself to a Peasant." You are to know that, after I left Apt and had set out on my journeying, I came upon a huge wagon which had been overturned and blocked the road diagonally. The peasant who stood beside it called out to me, begging me to help him with the wagon. I looked at the wagon. Truly, my arms are not without strength and the peasant seemed quite a man, too. But how were two men to lift up that enormous weight? "I cannot do it," I said. The other snarled at me. "You can," he cried, "but you're not willing." That struck me to the heart. We had some boards; we inserted them under the wagon and used all our strength in this act of leverage. The wagon stirred and rose and stood. We piled the hay on it again. The peasant passed his hand over the sides of the oxen who still trembled and panted. They began to draw. "Let me walk with you a while," I said. "Come right along, brother," he answered. We trod along together. "I would like to ask you something," I said. "Ask all you like, brother," he answered. "How did you happen to think," I asked him, "that I was unwilling to help?" "I thought of that," he replied, "because you said you could not help. No one knows whether he can do a thing until he has tried it." "But how did you happen to think," I questioned him again, "that I could do this thing?" "Oh that," he answered, "that just popped into my mind." "What do you mean by that?" "Ah, brother," he said, "what an insistent fellow you are. Very well, it popped into my mind, because you had been sent my way." "You will end by telling me that your wagon was upset in order that I might help you!" "Well of course, brother, what else?"' (Buber 1981, pp.32–3)

Martin Buber, and my mother (then Eva Schwarz), both left Germany in the 1930s; Buber departing for Jerusalem and my mother eventually for Australia. At that time, Australia encouraged immigration principally from Great Britain. However, a policy existed whereby resident citizens who were willing to sponsor, and financially support, relatives threatened by oppression in Europe could facilitate their entry into Australia. My mother continues to tell her story:

> Arnold Schwarz, my paternal grandfather, was the only one of seven brothers to stay in Germany. When the Franco-Prussian war ended in 1872, three brothers went to the United States of America. In 1879, Josef originally went to London, then Adelaide, and was the only one to keep his name as Schwarz. He was a metal worker in wrought iron and made the railings for numerous balconies of various well-known buildings, such as the King Edward, Old Melbourne and Great Britannia hotels, and for most of the pubs on the goldfields, such as Coolgardie, Boulder and Kalgoorlie. Unfortunately, on completion of the railings of the famous Palace Hotel in Kalgoorlie, the miners plied him with drink. He had 'one too many' and fell over the railings to his death. His grave is the only black marble one (Schwarz means black!!) in the old section of the Perth Jewish Cemetery. One brother went to Victoria, another to Queensland. In 1936–7, my parents searched for relatives in the USA, to no avail, so they advertised in all Australian States. The advertisement was noticed, in the *West Australian Judean* magazine, by a Mr. Solomon, who promptly contacted Albert Schwarz, the dentist, son of the late Josef. Albert's Catholic mother encouraged him to seek out his old school mate, John Curtin, Leader of the Opposition, who was to become Australia's wartime Labour Prime Minister, to ask for the entry permit. My father, who had been interned in Buchenwald in May 1938, was released in July when the permit arrived.

(Indeed, to this day, we have the letter, signed by John 'Black Jack' McEwen, a politician opposed to Labour values and countersigned by John Curtin, seeking the Schwarz's immigration into Australia).

> I had left Germany in 1936, to undertake some training as a nurse in London and a laboratory technician in Florence. We all met in Marseilles in August 1938 for our embarkation by boat to Australia. We held Services for Rosh Hashana and Yom Kippur, with about fifty people in attendance, mainly from 2nd and 3rd Class. To honour his 1st Class passengers, the Captain invited us, the Governor-General designate, Viscount Gowrie, and Lady Gowrie, and four other Jewish Australians to dine with him. Because it was the evening preceding Yom Kippur, he especially arranged for us all to eat at 5.00PM, well

before the Fast was to begin, and not the usual 7.30PM sitting. But two of the Australians came to dinner at the later time, dressed in fancy dress for the party celebrating our departure from Colombo, and so had to eat by themselves. For Sukkoth we even had a Sukkah on the 3rd Class deck and picked up fresh palm leaves to construct its roof, in Colombo! We travelled during the Czech Crisis. We took on troops in Malta, Port Said, Sudan and Aden to off-load them in Bombay. To travel in the black-out through the Red Sea was not much fun. In those days, the boats were not air-conditioned, only fans, so everyone used the decks. We arrived in Perth, Western Australia, on 18th October 1938. We were not aware of Albert Schwarz's change of religion until we arrived. Thus, what a surprise awaited us on our arrival at their home when, instead of the Mezzuzah on the front door, we saw a full-length picture of the "Sacred Heart' on the end-wall of their corridor. But it was the Catholic mother who had told her son Albert that Family comes first, that to let us perish in Germany would be a sin and thus a crime.

Backpage

The following story was told during a stage performance, in Melbourne in 1993, by the *Besht* tellers, and remains one of my favourites. I usually share it with clients towards the end of therapy. The therapeutic conversation is a creative process that encourages us to reflect on our lives and explore options for a different, more agreeable future. The story of Baal Shem Tov invites us to continue fashioning stories out of our lives and to pass them on to future generations, in the belief that even the meekest soul can compose a tale that is welcome at the Gates of Heaven.

The famous Rabbi Baal Shem Tov (the *Besht*), who lived in the early 18th century, heard that his community was facing a grave crisis. The *Besht* went into a forest, lit a fire and recited a prayer. God saw and heard all that the Rabbi did and He saved the community. In the next generation, the son of the *Besht* also heard that his community was threatened. He went into the forest and lit a fire but somehow could not remember the prayer. Nonetheless, God acknowledged what the son did and prevented the disaster that endangered the community. The grandson of the *Besht* learnt that once again the community was confronted with serious trouble. He went into the forest but had no knowledge of lighting the fire and the prayer was very far from his mind. Still, God saw and brought the community respite. Hardship, it seems, occurs in every generation and the *Besht's* great-grandson became aware of an imminent stress to the community. But this great-grandson did not know in which direction to walk to the forest, had not a clue about making the fire and the prayer was a very distant memory indeed. So the young man sat by a window in his house and told God how, in times of strife, his great-grandfather, Rabbi Baal Shem Tov, would go into the forest, light a fire and say a prayer…and God heard…and God spared the community. And do you want to know why? Because God loves good stories!

Appendix A
'Love, Pain and the Whole Damn Thing'

Poetry can be an effective framework within which clients and therapists can meet, a literary context within which to communicate our experiences. Poets attempt to convey what they are experiencing through the written word and invite readers to reflect on what they are experiencing as they read. I find it sometimes useful to invite clients either to compose their own verses or to share some of mine with them, so that, in reflecting on the lines together, we may open up a new area for discussion. Below is a collection of my poems, which endeavours to express some facets of human relating. The first eight poems might best be described as written 'in the blush of first love'. Obviously, I don't share the more erotic ones with clients (they were written for my own fun!) but I share poems such as 'Friendship' with couples who are deepening their intimacy. When couples are experiencing episodes of mismeeting, conflict and separation, Poems 9–14, 'Un-Coupling' and 'Communication Games', can be helpful in exploring some of the feelings clients may be experiencing but have difficulty in articulating. After separation comes a period of grieving and Poems 15–20, such as 'Hope-Lessening', 'Seasons' and 'Steel, Brick and Glass', can facilitate expression of the very real feelings of sadness, anger, confusion, void and despair that accompany loss. 'The Journey' and 'Homeward Bound' reflect eventual acceptance of changes that inevitably take place when either loss or reconciliation occurs. Following crises, when people acknowledge their emotional world in a more authentic manner, they may be more able to imagine the real of their partner's world; they may be able to invite their partner into this emotional world that they have newly discovered, to be included with their partner within an I–Thou position; they may be more able to respond to their partner's invitations to enter the partner's world. Poems 21–25 are about concert halls, beach holidays and lovely gardens, and people confirming their partnership as a mutual venture.

Courting:

1. Friendship[1]

Friendship is the meeting of two hearts,
The interchange of feelings, redefining
Of how two intimates relate. Unlike the refining
Of precious metals, with removal of unwanted parts,
The dross in our friends is accepted. Our rough, rude
Corners are not smoothed over, sculpted away,
But loved and understood. That is a friend's way.
We cherish our friends and accept their change in mood.
In friends we find ourselves. We complete
Ourselves and are larger than before.
We accept ourselves. We become more
Tolerant. We learn how others feel
And think, their pains and joys, the real,
The dishonest, the bitter – and the sweet.

2. A Passing Moment

We met. It was meant to be a passing moment,
Briefly encountering in a pleasant diversion of no lasting
Value. A minor interaction between mortals. A mere tasting
Of each other, not a fullsome meal. Having greeted, and spent
Some time together, I was to think on it
No more. I would let our dialogue go and move onward
To other events and places, progress without backward
Glance at where and when or with whom I had split.
Ah, how different! how delightful! the result of our contact,
For from the first we touched on deeper planes;
A yearning for connection established our friendship as fact.
We experienced each other's triumphs, disturbances, pains
And achievements; not underestimated or handled complacently
Were our many passing moments, shared in intimacy.

---

1   This poem was originally presented in Gunzburg 1993 p.328.

3. In a Quiet Encounter

Love's bond came from where? I did not seek
It and it appeared in an unexpected place;
In a quiet encounter, on a stranger's face,
Suddenly it was there. I tried to speak
My thoughts and found that my words were love.
I met you, shyly looked at you, and recognised
That touch and talk (I was surprised!)
Had grown into affection. We made a move
Away and found that our memories were of one another.
And when we came together to greet,
It was with warmth and welcome. To meet
And in our meetings keep our space;
For, loving friends, we knew our place
Was to love…not overwhelm each other.

4. Meeting With Words

I loved you not as Romeo loved Juliet,
Not all a buzz and full of passion's fire,
Not all-consumed by 'I must have you' desire,
With heaving loins and gropes and lover's sweat;
My regard for you kept its distance. We met with words.
Eating berries at Bulga Park, we touched each other's heart,
And nourished ourselves with remembrances when apart,
Of those good times that companionship affords.
Our bond developed in a special way, as an aid
To our growth, as an ease to our embattled souls.
It gave us comfort, warmth and peace. We laid
Our foundations for a mateship with longterm goals,
And we began to know ourselves. And when we reach our end,
When we contemplate our passage, we'll say: 'This was my friend'.

Coupling:

5. Cycles

Our relationship cycled, like Nature's changes,
With Wet Winter's morn and Summer's sweating noon,
Sol's heated glare and delicate pale of moon…
Yet our encounters were both subtle and extreme. Our exchanges
Of affection were both marvellous and moderate. We would kiss
With limbs all-clung, hung on each other's frames,
By passion driven, calling out erotic names,

Panting and heaving for satisfaction; and then suffer distress,
With sighs and thoughts of each other when apart! But our bond
Also contained such tenderness. We had contacts of quieter kind.
Like the gentle drift of bushland stream, our fond
Embrace and conversation involved a flow of mind
And emotions enjoined. Together, in sweet-swirling harmonies,
We shared ourselves within unique, yet entwined, destinies.

6. Reflections

Evening falls. An empty house, and I was alone,
Resting from the bustle of a day's work done,
Pondering on the speed at which swift hours had flown,
Listening to a record... Bach, in muted tone.
You were away at a meeting. I wondered if life treated you well?
Hoped that your day had passed and left you calm,
Kept you whole and integrated, and free from harm,
Trusted that you had rested, enjoying some still
Quiet moments within your busy routine. Tonight was not ours.
Other commitments kept us apart, and out of touch;
So I spent my evening softly, filling my leisure hours
With music and pleasant memories, warm feelings of how much
I valued your presence when we were together. Not for me to mourn
Those times we could not have, but patiently to await another dawn.

7. Strokes of Delight

A poem for pleasure...let me be the strokes of delight,
Tracing your shapely form and with my firmness pressed
Within your delicious softness, hands warmly cupping breasts
Like pomegranates, journey with you passionately to Heaven's height;
These joys are ours; our relationship affords us this...
But I want also to love you with words and penetrate deep
Into your soul, giving you a dreamer's sleep
With images of being upheld and dearly valued. Let kiss
And caress conveyed in verses complement lover's thrust.
Let my sonnets affirm our bond, cement our union;
Let me pledge a partnership of support and nourishment shared;
I will promise commitment leading to lifelong communion,
Treasured by us both. There you have it, love...unspared
Are my expressions, telling them to you openly as I must.

8. Serenade

A poem for quieter mode...the fanfare has played.
Interwoven harmonious themes have risen to crescendo,
Thumped out their climactic chords and, satisfied, let go.
My experiences, urgent for utterance, are made public, displayed
As musical rhythms within the lines on these pages.
Music, script and emotions are all blended as one,
Feelings verbalized, songs that needed to be sung,
And sonnets that illustrate my inner world within the stages
Of our relationship. There is often a lively tempo with mood
Uplifted. Rarely is there sadness and clouded despair,
Mostly comfort and calm acceptance. These are good
Times that we both share quite free from care;
Delightful tunes flow within me. O let them never end,
These serenades that play for you, my beloved friend.

Un-Coupling:

9.

Not talking
kept us together.

What was not said
was understood
to be unspeakable.

When we started
timorously
to tell each other
how it was for us,
we split.

Now, well divorced,
we converse continuously,
bitter words spat out,
our feelings shared.

10.

Communication games...
names spoken
about how things are not
with us.

Words masking
what we feel.

Too difficult for us
to tolerate
too much that is real.

11.

Coming closer,
with fears, stammering,
an awkward pause,
then withdrawal, and distance;
calm now, no cause
for alarm...
Again an approach,
with anxieties abundant,
a flare of temper,
then tantrums, and a slamming door;
apart now, all settled...
with a glance over my shoulder
at the absence in your chair.

12.

What now?
Such a face!
Quickly,
to avoid discovering what it means,
without words,
without ever a suggestion
of inner turmoil,
mine or hers.
To reinstate order
abruptly, effectively,
without ever knowing
the 'why' of such a face...

13.

A frown, fists clenched,
with words that do not match her mood,
She wishes to be believed.

'I love you' (with such a look?)
Her look, with: 'Honey, you know I do!'

She scarcely comprehends
The disjointedness of her communications
and my unease.

Her look is no love…
And love? Never with those looks!
Be dutiful,
Accept her statements,
Be deceived!

14.

Talking tattle,
marital prattle,
weather hopeful, Mrs. Bull's
new shoes all shiny, spiny
urchins eating reefs and beef
more costly, mostly gays and drugs
in Sydney, kidney pie and beans
for dinner, winners are 'the Saints' (St. Kilda),
Hilda gone to bed forlorn,
sworn is the jury in the dingo trial,
and vile crime is prime time on T.V.,
See that Charlie's son got shot?
What bloody rot! Bereft, I left!

Grieving:

15. Emptiness

Loneliness lingers beneath the rooftops.
Concrete slabs of orange, gray and green,
The shingles shelter no persons within.

They cover no gentle contact between lovers,
No conversations, no interactions.

In the houses without people
The rooms are bare
Save for chairs, a sofa, some tables,
And stairways leading up to shadowy attics,
further emptiness.

Their occupants are employed elsewhere;
Drinking their coffee, commuting
Alone, without ever knowing
The inner-world of their others; isolated, earning

Their living without ever learning
The wherefore of each other.

At day's dreary end,
Under the rooftops they gather,
Family members without ever meeting,
From workplace lethargy to domestic lassitude,
Nurtured by the media presenter,
They collect, and keep their distance
As best as they can.

16. Hope-Lessening

In my mind, a raging
Like winds whipping grains on a sandy shore
Against stinging legs. And I wish I could change
Those gusts to peaceful whispers once more.

In my limbs, an aging
And with that growing old comes black despair,
A lessening of hope that ancient wounds will heal,
No lessening of the anxieties that I bear.

In my living, a caging
Within a cell and no way out, no passage
To future fancies, no exit to a lighter existence,
No option for movement from shadows to centre stage.

And in my performance, played out
Is my song, unstrung is my bow, untuned
My fiddle, with melodies faded away
to silence…and a soulful deathmask assumed.

17. Seasons

Autumn is not sadness. Red-berried branch and twig fallen,
Brown leaf crushed on parkland grass do not signal
Death and decay, rather pause in Nature's cycle;
Fruits distended with ripe flesh, drooped golden
Blooms about to drop do not herald an end
To life, merely a slowing in organic process;
Autumn leads not to gravestone, rather Winter recess,
A time for rest where hearts heal and breaks mend.
So is my current existence. I wonder at the reason
I find myself disconsolate, alone. I ask:' Why me?
Am I the foolish one to find myself in the season
Of my discontent?' Winter's chill has come early

For me. Why the discomfort I can never fully know.
Mine is to bide Winter-time, to heal and grow.

Acceptance:

18. The Journey[2]

I had a vision that was not purely fancy;
Above the world I hovered as a spirit
Free from the binds of 'this all too solid flesh'
And from my vantage point was able to observe
A trail below me well-covered with brown dirt;
A winding path that wavered in its width,
Here large enough for a human form to pass,
There narrowed, stopping passage of all but smallest
Creatures. Rocks rough-hewn by winter's frosty
Morn lay strewn, gray granite cracked and worn;
Scattered stones and tufts of withered grass,
And shiny pieces of broken glass. Wasps
And mayflies flew there, gumtrees drooped, dried
Bushes scratched the naked legs of travellers
Passing along who paused to wince. The sun
Shone down and raised a sweat on necks and backs,
Moist patches spread on shorts and shirts. All sorts
Of hats were worn to cover aching heads from heat.
A motley of shapes and sizes trekked that track;
Young lads who wandered off into the scrub
Were called by snarling mothers: 'Andrew, don't you
Go too far!' The men came stumbling, bruising
Knees and cursing softly, hoping for a breeze
To cool them down; the women wilting, fumbling
With anxious fingers, fiddling in bags for tissues
To wipe the plump, wet cheeks of babes; the grizzle
Of a fallen toddler, and tousle-haired sisters singing
Gaily a nursery rhyme, hands held. And as this multitude
Proceeded on their journey, the bushland sounded
With their conversations of money and friendships and leisure,
With good-humoured chuckles, chatting and moans of ill-temper,
Young lover's snippets and dreary whistles of boredom.
Incessantly, inexorably, the flow of persons continued
Along this well-worked route that led to forests afar.

---

2   This poem was originally presented in Gunzburg 1993, pp.377–8.

Sometimes they happened upon a stagnant pool
Where they would dip their feet and, with wet kerchief
On brow, would soothe their fevers. Occasionally running
Streams provided drink and, if their luck was fair,
Blackberries were there to eat. When there was shade
They took it, otherwise enduring harsh open spaces
With resignation and the chance of a better track ahead.
They progressed as best as they knew how with whatever
Skills they possessed; some faltered, halting on the way,
Then moving on, others determined to go no further,
But for all, there was no possibility of retreat,
No option for return;
For this was their only journey,
It was their life.

19. Steel, Brick and Glass

Rocks are impervious to pain. Hills do not feel
The sting of brutish life. They stand throughout Time
As enduring memorials to Nature's forces, sublime
Monuments to creative grandeur. Buildings of steel,
Brick and glass are oblivious to human interaction.
They last for decades, unmindful of those who pass through
Their doors, heedless of when and where and who
Are industrious within; cold monoliths, unconcerned with action
Of Mortals. Not so with the World of Experience. It spans
A few years, knows joy, tears, discomfort, the touch
Of lips soft-pressed, the hug of consolation, hands
Held gently, the tender phrase: 'I love you much'.
It recognises Distance, is conscious of Finite Time,
Affirming not uncaring Nature, but Love as its theme.

20. Homeward Bound
(written on a Nullabor coach ride)

Windswept plain, what stories do you tell?
Travellers sweating their tiresome passage on aching foot,
Gay parrots wending their way on high and the rotten smell
Of wallabies killed by speeding traffic on the highway. A boot,
A tire and a rusting can are left as obscenities
By those who use and dispose. in the heat of the day
Our coach stops by a bullet-pocked sign which reads: 'Amenities
Ahead'. Some passengers alight and stretch, others stay
inside and nibble. Some sleep, some keep conversing

As if their journey's cessation was of no great matter.
We commence again, our cylinders grinding, our vehicle traversing
An unswerving bitumen strip. Now music, and the natter
Of our coach-captain: 'Here is a mountain, there an historic mound',
And I with different thoughts and emotions; homeward, bound.

Reconciliation:

21. St. Kilda Botannical Gardens

I can always go 'home' to the flowers;
When world-weary cares rest heavily on shoulder,
When irksome thoughts fill working hours
With well-meant intentions and obsessions that smoulder,
I cease every labour, and exit my room
To visit a vision that bejewels my street;
Through gates always partially open I stroll, and am home.
There, palm trees spreading green fans, sweet
Scents and colours ablaze in the sun await
Me...my soul is uplifted, my inner aches abate,
I let loose tense limbs, shedding chains, and am free;
At one with the One, bloomed anew: I am me.

22. Farewell, the Tall Ships

(5/1/88: written when the sailing vessels of many nations visited
Melbourne during Australia's Bicentennial celebrations)

Windblown folds in sails unfurled,
Spray against bows that slice through foam;
Blue skies above us with cloud-wisps curled
In the distance...the tall ships are sailing home.

Masts lancing upward pull rigging taught,
With ropes tugged tight and anchors aweigh;
Barques and brigantines, boats of all sort
Are grouped on the bay...the tall ships are away.

And when shall we view such grandeur again?
We who observe them in wonder, and cheer;
When will we sight the likes of such men
And women who graced us with their presence this year?

Never again, for this was unique, an event
That will not be repeated, that is classified: 'No more';
And our dreams will remind us of the fleet that was sent
By the world cross great waters to dance at our door.

23. Rhapsody In Blue
(conceived during a performance at the Melbourne Concert Hall)

The clarinet's languid tones scale upward,
Caressing the sound-shells hanging from the roof,
Then downward glide to the aisles. We, the audience
Who sit beneath the shells are spellbound by the notes,
Quite still, breaths held. Now the pianist begins,
With slender fingers rippling across the keys, enchanting us.
Her eyes catch the conductor's glance.
They exchange knowing looks that bind them...
And so are we, their listeners,
Bound by their loving performances, by their harmonies
Blended as one...

Rhapsodies in blue, you woo me,
Setting my spirit and fancies free,
Stirring the primitive passions within,
Opening a wild-world that beckons me in...

Brass and woodwinds spit, stretched hide and strings
Vibrate together; swirls of crescendo,
Noisy fanfares, trills and blistering chords
Resound, then pause...and applause echoes all around.

24. Childer's Cove Holiday
(written during a Summer's holiday at the beach with my family)

Breaking wave on rock-face fallen,
Fossil crab in sand discovered,
Shells on shore and seaweeds swollen,
Seagull's form above us, hovered;
Caves in limestone, cool and shaded,
Swimmers splashing, children shouting,
Daughters climbing cliffs unaided,
In the distance, dolphins spouting;
Sun on shoulder, warm and soothing,
Spouse beside me resting, graceful,
Sand on nose tip, cute, amusing:
Thanks to God for lives not wasted.

25. *To a Wife*

Moments of closeness so precious
That my lips cannot express
Our emotions intertwining, treasured
Moments of tenderness...
And when apart, not space,
But an essence remains with me;
In mind I picture your lovely face,
In distance, my thoughts are coupled with thee.

Appendix B[1]

Some useful questions to facilitate the therapeutic conversation

1. Questions that encourage *meeting* between therapists and their clients, and that invite clients to participate within a *genuine dialogue*:

> How did you get to hear of me?
>
> How do you come to be here?
>
> What is happening with you?
>
> What is troubling you?
>
> What are your struggles?
>
> What are you stuck with?
>
> Which area of stress most bothers you?
>
> How might I be of help to you?
>
> How might I best help your family?
>
> How could things be different for you?
>
> Would you write a few lines (draw a picture, compose a poem or song) for the next session, describing what it is like for you at the moment?
>
> Would your partner, family come to a future session of therapy with you?
>
> Why do you think I asked you to come here with your Mum/Dad today?

2. Questions that enable therapists to *imagine the real* of their clients' world, and that *include* clients and therapists within the therapeutic conversation:

> When did you first feel like this?
>
> What was happening at the time?
>
> Where did you learn to do that?
>
> Where did that come from?
>
> What do you think that means?

---

1   A number of these questions were included in Gunzburg and Stewart 1994, pp.290–9.

Would you put your feelings down on paper?

What is your favourite piece of music, film, play, book, etc?

Could your problem be described by drawing it as a shape? What size and colour is it? How could you protect yourself from it?

Imagining the real of the client's family of origin

(a) Relating to family expectations:

What role do you think you played in the family in which you grew up?

What unreasonable expectation of your family of origin is most bothersome to you?

Who, of all those persons in your family of origin, was there to tend to your youthful needs adequately and appropriately? How have you been able to cope with the demands and competition within your original family?

Where was the opportunity for privacy and adolescent reflection in your family of origin?

Were many of the expectations within your family of origin geared towards the advancement of men leaving little time for leisure and fun?

Did your mother invite you, at an early age, to be her partner against the apparent patriarchal attitudes of the men in the family? Has your mother written a script for you, one of helplessness, and one that reflects her own helplessness? What would have to happen for you to retire from this role of being your mother's partner against the oppression of women by the men, and to write your own script?

Is there a family tradition of emotional deprivation by the men within your family?

Was this one of the reasons that one parent was so angry at the other? Did one parent slot the other into a subordinate role? How much of your mother's deprivation and abuse of you do you think was influenced by her husband's criminal violations of her?

Have you internalized the critical part of one parent and partnered an authoritarian person very much like the other parent? Is this contributing to your inner conflict?

(b) Relating to parental separation:

Did your parents, in parting when you were young, sensitize you to the risks and possible losses inherent in intimate relationships?

Was one parent overcome with grief when the separation occurred? Perhaps this parent felt immobilized and needed your young strength to help him/her succeed?

Would things have been better/worse if your parents had parted during your infancy?

(c) Relating to abuse within the family:

Did your family, frustrated by your parent's alcohol abuse, agree to a secret agenda not to comment about it?

Do you feel that your sexually abusing parent (sibling) has poisoned you?

What sort of father would you have liked to have had?

Imagining the real of the client's current intimacies

(a) Relating to patriarchy:

Do the men in your life all follow patriarchal scripts that allow them to define their sense of masculinity to the disadvantage of their female partners?

Do you think that your partner is inherently evil or is he following a well-learned patriarchal script?

(b) Relating to the quality of the intimacy:

What would have to happen to let each other know that you cared about each other?

What do you value about each other?

Do you want to continue your relationship?

Does God demand impossible standards? rigid roles? lack of autonomy and initiative? denial of sexual intimacy where respect and liking is present between partners?

Do you think that you are treating your partner similarly to the way one of your parents treated the other?

Do you think that you married your partner to gain some of the emotional nourishment that you had been denied earlier on?

If you keep yourself so fired up, is your partner liable to send off a heat-seeking missile and blow you out of the sky?

Is your ex-partner testing your gallantry? Is she inviting you on a holiday to check if you are able to behave decently in those circumstances, then, having passed the test, does she set you up to do battle with her new boyfriend?

Are your panic attacks and headaches and neck pains more to do with cementing your relationship to your partner, than with your work?

Is your partner's current abusive behaviour consistent with wanting a more rewarding relationship?

Is your partner's behaviour (drinking, leaving), a response to your actions, or is he/she responsible for his/her own actions and choices?

What is it specifically that troubles you about your relationship with your partner?

Why did you originally choose each other as partners?

How can you assess your partner's ability to make commitment to an intimacy?

Do you interpret your partner's wishes for 'closeness' as 'clinging'?

What shared experiences might continue to nourish you?

How can you intrigue your partner into a different and more rewarding kind of encounter?

How can you both find your own roots within your relationship?

How might you achieve mutuality and equity in your negotiations with your partner?

How can you learn to compete successfully with your partner?

How can you ask for what you want without feeling guilty?

Are your arguments involving you with each other or creating distance?

Is it easier to argue with your partner than to be sad?

Have you been working under such duress that there has been little time for fun?

Have all your energies gone into parenting?

Are some of your current emotions grief for lost moments, opportunities for intimacy, peace of mind growth?

Is your relationship another child, to be nurtured into growth?

(c) Relating to affairs:

Is your affair part of your search for happiness? Are there less painful ways to achieve the fulfillment that you seek? What would happen if you did tell your partner about your affair?

Have you lost the 'specialness' within your marriage and sought it with your lover instead?

Do the triangular relationships within which you live prevent you from gaining the information you need to know before making a couples commitment?

Do you believe that you will ever maintain a monogamous relationship?

How can you make a permanent and enduring commitment to a partner?

Should you proceed with reconciliation with your former partner, or follow a future with your new friend?

If you were prepared to invite your former partner or your new friend to therapy, which one would attend?

Should you be residing with your former partner, offering him/her false hope, if you have definitely decided to leave?

Did you have an affair to learn new information and bring this into your primary intimacy?

Was your affair a rebellion against your parents' values? What would have happened if you had taken a lover of different faith to yours?

Do you expect Divine retribution for your adultery?

What would happen if you carried out your one-night homosexual affair and found that you really liked the experience better than your current partner?

What will your partner have to do now, after his/her affair, to restore your trust?

How can your sense of 'belonging' in your relationship now be restored after her/his affair?

(d) Relating to separation:

Are you trying to preserve the ideal of an intact family at the risk of bodily injury?

How would you benefit from separation?

Over what aspects of the past relationship would you grieve?

What memories would you take with you to nourish your future?

What 'unspeakable things' have you really done to drive your former partner away?

Is your former partner behaving with goodwill towards your family?

Is your former partner being respectful, and sensitive to the needs of other family members?

Is there so much fighting all the time in the family, to make sure that everyone is getting a fair share of the attention?

What would your parents do if you pushed them just that bit too far?

Do you (children) feel confident about reaching adulthood? Is it worthwhile to grow to adulthood, with all the struggles that you have already witnessed within your families? Is adulthood all hard work and sorrows, with little fun and rewards?

Are you still mourning the loss of your marriage and displacing the anger of your grief onto your children? Is your anger a way of contacting your children?

Are you fearful that Mum and Dad might divorce?

Do you know the reason for your parents' separation?

Are you, a son, grieving your parents' divorce, and is anger the only way permitted to men to express their grief within our society? Is your father also grieving his divorce, and is his withdrawal from you his way of avoiding the pain of expressing his own sadness?

Is your family better or worse since the separation?

Do you see the parent who lives away regularly on access? Do you want to? Does the parent who lives away know that you want to see them?

Do you think that you drove Mum or Dad away? If you had behaved better, might they might have stayed together? Do you feel it is your fault that they have separated?

Do you think that some of the emotions that you feel because one parent blamed you for the other parent leaving have become stuck inside of you, and are not able to get out?

Do you believe that your custodial parent is committed to caring for you until adulthood?

Did you really tell such a lie, or did you express to others just how bad it felt for you to be rejected by your partner?

Imagining the real of the client's current emotional world

(a) Relating to the social world:

Perhaps the jeering of your school mates encouraged you to want to be inconspicuous? I guess you are most comfortable when you are the invisible man. How can you be imperceptible with your two lively friends around you?

Is your struggle similar to that which this person experienced? Do you know how to ask for what you want?

Can the friends' voices that you hear in your head be regarded as advisers, offering you wise counsel?

Who were the voices that guided you when you were young? Are you giving up on your life?

What qualities do you remember of those people who most influenced you during your teen years? What if you were to arrange a celebration? Which qualities of those people would she invite along?

Will you let me arrange for the children to go into foster care for the weekend, and find a trusted friend available to come and stay with you so that you can get some rest?

Will your foster family respect expression of your feelings?

(b) Relating to self perceptions and inner feelings:

Are you a bit of a perfectionist?

Are you blaming the past for your current struggles?

Is that why you are so scared, and vomiting? Is there so much sick feeling inside you, that once started, you may never stop?

Is some of your anger now inwardly channelled and contributing to your low spirits?

Would you list the ways that you have tried to tackle your 'emptiness'?

Does your fear of going mad seem like madness itself?

Would you write a conversation with your rage: what is it doing for you? What would happen if you became less forceful? How can you and your rage strike a bargain so that you do not have to drink, either for comfort or to temper your anger?

(c) Relating to illness and death:

What if your illness is not caused by your quarrels with your family? What if it is bad luck that you have now got this disease, and your anger at your family is getting in the way of any chance of reconciliation that you might have with them before you die?

What do you hope for in the time left to you?

Are you hopeful of something better?

Would you write a letter to the 'healthy person you were' saying goodbye?

How will you manage at your partner's funeral?

Do you need to let your child experience the privacy of his grief for his deceased parent?

What will happen if you do carry out your plans to suicide?

Does the presence of your parent's ghost now plague you with panicky feelings, headaches and muscle tensions?

Do you think that your child's death was a sort of punishment?

(d) Relating to professional abuse:

How does your client with whom you are professionally involved and having an affair feel? Will you stop this professional abuse? Will you make a commitment not to professionally abuse your clients in the future? What will life be like if you maintain your commitment not to professionally abuse your clients? How will you redress your professional abuse of your clients?

3. Questions that invite clients to *confirm* themselves.

Confirming the self

What will it be like for you when life is better?

What is happening now that life is better?

Was there ever a time when life was better?

Were there people in the past who helped life to be better?

Are they available to you now?

If, by magic, you woke up, and life was better, how would you know?

What character from a film, book, opera, etc, would you most like to be like?

If you wanted to change your name, which one would you choose?

What bridges are there to cross for you to succeed in your search for a fulfilling life?

When do you think that your wandering will come to an end and you will 'be at home'?

Will you take some time out to do a relaxation exercise?

Will you imagine a different future?

What messages of self-esteem will you give to yourself?

How will you take charge of your life?

How will you ask for what you want more effectively?

What will have to happen for you to feel cherished again?

How will you become the central character in a script of your own choosing?

What decisions do you need to discover a more authentic lifestyle?

What will it be like when you are able to interpret your own dreams, rather than follow an external authority's guide to their meaning?

Will you make a commitment to contest any person who attempts to abuse you?

Will you write a letter contesting your parent's/ partner's abuse, deprivation, etc?

Will you compose a letter to your abusive relative and tell him/her what you have just told to me?

Will you take some time out to draw your experiences of the rape?

Will you write a conversation with your grieving self, who has missed out on many nourishing moments within your original family?

Will you write a letter to your internal saboteur, delivering a K. O. blow, and telling your saboteur that you do have rights?'

Will you compose a self-advertisement for the next session?

Will you list ten ways to boost your confidence when feeling low?

Will you make a list of things that you want to achieve in your life?

Will you make a list of your needs now?

Will you consider the difference between what you need in life and what you want?

Will you write a description of what it means to be an adequate person?

Will you use your courage to become your own person, and leave the family territory to fight the oppression by men against women on your own terms? Will you list some ways of reaching out to the world outside your family and imagine what your life might be like in five years time?

Will you seek safety in a life of your own, perhaps with the support of friends, rather than in an abusive primary relationship?

Will you gather the necessary information you need to know to pursue a career in…?

How will you seek personal integration and fulfillment?

Will you write a conversation with your developing self, who wishes to explore more rewarding directions for the future?

Will you script a conversation with Madonna, seeking advice from her on how to mould personality out of confusion?

Will the 'caring person' inside you compose a conversation with the 'crying person' inside you and offer her comfort and guidance? Will you continue to ask the 'wise person' how she/he will guide the 'crying person'?

Will you write a short essay describing what it means for you to keep a kosher kitchen?'

Will you compose a list of some of the positive qualities that your parents have given you, qualities which now affirm you and help you to know who you are?

How will you, a terminally ill person, be productive in the time left? How will you battle against all odds? How will you cheat death? How will creativity arise out of decay? How will you give towards the future? How will you return to your roots? How will you achieve belonging and permanence?

Will you write a letter to God to find out why He has said 'No!' to you so often?

Will you compose a list of qualities that you, your former partner, and your new friend have contributed to your relationships?

Will you draw a 'rogues gallery' of all the partners who have mistreated you in the past?

Will you write a letter to your 'internal critic' and find out what it wants of you?

Will you plan a time schedule and budget for separation?

Will you contest your former partner's 'guilt hooks' and vengeful remarks?

Will you contact your former partner, who broke off your relationship unilaterally, and clarify the reasons as to why he/she acted in this way?

Will you make a specific list of ten curses to fall upon your former partner?

Will you compose a few lines for your Valentine's card to let your former partner know that she/he is indeed loved, without raising any false hopes for the future?

Will you look at some photographs of your deceased partner, prepare a list of your memories, and choose those that you want to keep secret and those that you might reveal?

Will you bring some of your deceased parent's drawings to the next session?

Will you write yourself a letter from your deceased partner advising you on how to cope in this difficult situation?

Will you draw a picture in memory of your partner's beloved deceased pet?

Will you re-dream the scene of your relative's death and visualize a different ending?

Will you visit to your relative's grave and say goodbye?

Will your story prove to be a way of rehearsing for the future, exploring what optimism and hope lies in the direction ahead?

What will it feel like when you are truly contented?

What aspect of therapy has been most helpful to you?

Confirming the family:

> Will you make a commitment not to abuse your partner or child in the future?
>
> Will you write a Commitment of Non-Abuse, Certificate of Non-Humiliation, etc, towards your partner or child?
>
> What will life be like if you maintain your commitment not to abuse your partner or child?
>
> Will you write a description of what responsibility means to you and how you can help the person you abused grow away from your violation of her?
>
> Will you write a description of how the person you abused feels? Will you continue to live apart from the family to maintain the safety of the person you abused?
>
> What ordinary activities might you participate in with the family to restore stability?
>
> Now that your children are growing into young adulthood, will you, who has been their custodial parent for all these years, find a more appropriate way of connecting with them (other than dumping your anger onto them) so that you can all share your emotional struggles with each other? Will you start sharing some details of the family's finances with them so that they can help prepare a budget? Will you all hold a Family Annual General meeting to discuss your future direction?
>
> Now that the family has confronted your uncle about his sexual abuses of you and your cousins, will you and your relatives arrange 'safety meetings', ensuring that the more vulnerable family members are protected?

Confirming the couple:

> Will you talk to your partner about your future dreams together?
>
> Will you both do something for next session?
>
> Will you try together to identify some of the trigger points at which you start quarrelling?
>
> Will you turn your words into praise for your partner's victories whenever he holds back from violence, rather than reminding your partner of those times he has lashed out?
>
> Will you draw the demons that you see within each other and experience within yourselves when you are angry?
>
> Will you both draw some pictures of the monsters that are disturbing your peace?

Will you compare and contrast the negative qualities of the 'old (Hugo)' of earlier years and the 'new (Hugo)' of present times and monitor what changes have occurred?

Will you compare and contrast the positive qualities between the 'old friendship' and the 'new friendship' so that you can both measure the triumphs that you have achieved together with the passage of time?

Will you write the pro's and con's of continuing a relationship with your partner?

Will you remember back to the time you were courting, and think about what you had hoped for at the beginning of your acquaintance?

Will you both sit down together and negotiate a Contract of Reconciliation?

Will you work towards making your relationship 'special' watching a video together, taking a night out for pizza and coffee, or going for a walk in the park?

Will you write to your parent describing how you are experiencing your relationship with your partner differently to the one you had with your parent?

Will you write an essay describing the struggle within your relationships?

Will you both write a bill of divorce from your parents/in-laws for the next session?

Will you trust your partner enough to organize a spontaneous weekend entertainment without your partner knowing what it is beforehand?

Will you give each other massage?

Will you plan an hour a week 'not being nasty' to each other?

Will you make a list of what is going right for you?

Will the two of you do a trade? Would you…?

Will you be prepared to experiment together as to just how you might achieve closeness and permanency within your relationship?

Will you do some nice things for each other, and see if each of you notices what the other person does?

Will you both consider some ways to fire up your match?

Will you reverse roles?

Will you consider what sacrifices you are prepared to make for each other's comfort, safety and fun?

Will you take yourselves out for a meal to celebrate raising your off-spring to adulthood and discuss if their is 'life after the children'?

Will you prepare yourself a special meal, a treat, and whilst eating it, occasionally feed one another a tasty morsel?

Will you continue to plan a direction that offers safety for you both?

Confirming parenting:

Will you protect your child from abuse?

Will you find out the telephone number of a refuge where you and your child can go if threatened with further abuse?

Will you organize a Gold Star Chart: if your children keep the dining-room, lounge, hallways clean of their rubbish five days each week, will you award them a silver star? If they keep those areas tidy three weeks each month, will you give them a gold star? For two months and two gold stars in a row, will you give them a special treat?

Will you take some time out together to spend with your children?

Will you take your children out to a restaurant and discuss how you all experience the problem?

Will you (the father) spend an hour's 'caring time' with your children, giving them some of the company that they might be wanting?

Will you (the father) take your child to the general practitioner for his/her next checkup?

Will you discuss the issue of whether you are to have children or not?

Will the two of you sit down, for a couple of hours each week, and talk about how one of you could support the other in the parenting of the other's children?

Will you and your adopted child go out for coffee one evening and discuss what you want from each other?

Will you list the happy times that you do remember spending with your adopted child?

Will you hold a special dinner to welcome your new foster-child?

Confirming the children:

Will your parent protect you from further abuse?

What has to happen so that you can now feel safe?

Do you think that the person who abused you can change? Can this person become responsible? Do you know what this person is doing to learn responsibility?

Will you arrange a 'fun activity' together with Mum and Dad, and spend one hour caring time with them each week to do it?

Will you read this story during a quiet moment with your parent and let me know your opinion of it?

Will you negotiate with your parents to arrange a weekend to go over and sleep at a friend's house?

Will you, the child who throws tantrums, draw a picture of your temper for a subsequent session, with the eventual aim of putting it in a 'temper box', and, with the encouragement of other family members, helping you to contain it in there?

Will you, a son, let your father know some of the sadness that underlies your anger? Will you invite your father to a session of therapy to discuss some 'men's stuff'?

Will you do a sketch of the family as you see them?

Will you plan a special treat for your adopting parent, something really subtle, and see if your parent detects it?

Will you compose a poem for your foster family describing how you feel about them?

Will you furnish your new bedroom, in your foster parents' home, to your own unique style?

(This list is by no means to be considered complete! Readers are encouraged to contemplate the questions and to generate new queries that invite meeting, genuine dialogue, imagining the real, inclusion and confirmation).

Glossary

Amidah – a prayer said standing, and in silence.

Baruch Haba – Blessed be those who come, traditional Jewish prayer.

Besht – acronym for Baal Shem Tov.

Ellul – the last month in the Jewish calendar.

Hasidim – Religious Jews who worship God through joyous prayer, singing, dancing and story-telling.

Klaus – refuge, hermitage.

Kol Nidrei – prayer that opens the Day of Atonement.

L'Hayyim – to (a good) life, traditional Jewish toast when drinking alcoholic beverages.

L'Hitraot – farewell, see you again sometime.

L'Shana Tova Tikatevi – (to females), A Happy new Year and may you be inscribed in the Book of Life. The corresponding greeting to males is L'Shana Tova Tikatevu.

Menschen – decent human beings

Mezzuzah – prayer box to be found on the right hand doorpost (as one enters) of Jewish homes. It contains written words of the Shema.

Pesach – Passover

Rosh Hashana – the Jewish New Year

Shabbat – the Sabbath, which occurs Jews every Saturday

Shalom – traditional Jewish greeting, meaning 'Peace'.

Shema – the quintessential Jewish declaration of faith: Hear, O Israel, the Lord our G-d, the Lord is One.

Shofar – a ram's horn trumpet, traditionally blown to sound an alarm, and to close the Day of Atonement.

Synagogue – Jewish house of prayer.

Sukkoth – the Feast of Tabernacles, a harvest festival occurring soon after the Day of Atonement, which celebrates the gathering of fruits from the fields in Israel.

Sukkah – a temporary booth, or tabernacle, built with a roof of green leaves and decorated with fruit and nuts. Observant Jews celebrate the eight days of Sukkoth by praying, eating, and even sleeping, in the Sukkah.

Tabernacle – sukkah (see above).

Talmud Torahs – religious Jewish student colleges.

Ten Days – there are traditionally ten days which are more favourable for repentance between, and including, Jewish New Year and the Day of Atonement.

Tishri – the first month in the Jewish calendar.

Torah – scrolls of parchment on which are written the Five Books of Moses; also called the 'Pentateuch'.

Yom Kippur – the Day of Atonement, a Fast Day for observant Jews.

Zaddikim – literally, 'righteous ones', but usually the leaders of the Hasidim, that is the late Lubavitcher Rebbe, Menahem Mendel Schneerson of New York. Zaddik is singular of Zaddikim.

Bibliography

Ackerman, N. (1958) *The Psychodynamics of Family Life.* New York: Basic Books.

Barron, F. (1968) *Creativity and Personal Freedom.* London: Van Nostrand.

Ben Asher, N. (1979) *Jewish Encyclopaedia.* New York: Shengold Publishers.

Buber, M. (1947) *Tales of the Hasidim.* New York: Schoken Books.

Buber, M. (1948) *Israel and the World. Essays in a Time of Crisis.* New York: Schocken Books.

Buber, M. (1958) *I and Thou.* 2nd edn. trans. by R.G. Smith. New York: Scribner's Son.

Buber, M. (1965) *The Knowledge of Man, A Philosophy of the Interhuman.* trans. by M. Friedman and R.G. Smith. New York: Harper and Row.

Buber, M. (1973) *Meetings.* LaSalle, IL: Open Court.

Buber, M. (1981) *For the Sake of Heaven, A Chronicle.* Translated by Ludwig Lewisohn. New York: Atheneum.

Courtney, B. (1989) *The Power of One.* Australia: Mandarin.

De Bono, E. (1970) *Lateral Thinking: A Textbook of Creativity.* New York: Harper and Row.

Edelstein, G. (1981) *Trauma, Trance and Transformation.* New York: Brunner-Mazel.

Ellis, A. (1987) *The Practice of Rational-Emotive Therapy.* New York: Springer.

Erikson, E. (1968) *Identity, Youth and Crisis.* New York: Norton.

Frankl, V. (1970) *Man's Search for Meaning.* New York: Touchstone.

Freud, S. (1960) *A General Introduction to Psychoanalysis.* New York: Washington Square Press.

Friedman, M. (1960) *Martin Buber: The Life of Dialogue.* New York: Harper and Row.

Friedman, M. (1985) *The Healing Dialogue in Psychotherapy.* New York: Jason Aronson.

Fromm, E. (1957) *The Art of Loving.* London: George Allen & Unwin.

Getzels, J.W. (1962) *Creativity and Intelligence with Gifted Students.* New York: Wiley.

Gunzburg, J.C. (1991) *The Family Counselling Casebook.* Sydney: McGraw-Hill.

Gunzburg, J.C. (1993) *Unresolved Grief: A Practical Multicultural Approach for Health Practitioners.* London: Chapman and Hall.

Gunzburg, J.C. (1994) 'What works?: Therapeutic experience with grieving clients.' *Journal of Family Therapy 16,* 2.

Gunzburg, J.C. and Stewart, W. (1994) *The Grief Counselling Casebook: A Student's Guide to Unresolved Grief.* London: Chapman and Hall.

Haley, J. (1973) *Uncommon Therapy: The Techniques of Milton H. Erickson.* New York: Norton.

Haley, J. (1984) *Problem Solving Therapy*. New York: Harper and Row.

Haley, J. (ed) (1985) *Conversations with Milton H. Erickson MD. Volume 2, Changing Couples*. New York: Triangle Press.

Jacobi, J. (1973) *The Psychology of C.J. Jung*. Newhaven: Yale University Press.

Jenkins, A, (1990) *Invitations to Responsibility: The Therapeutic Engagement of Men who are Violent and Abusive*. Adelaide: Dulwich Centre Publications.

Laing, R. (1965) *The Divided Self*. New York; Penguin.

Leupnitz, D.A. (1988) *The Family Interpreted: Feminist Theory in Clinical Practice*. New York: Basic Books.

Maslow, A. (1968) *Towards a Psychology of Being*. Princeton, New Jersey: Van Nostrand Reinhold.

May, R. (1970) *Symbolism, Religion, and Literature*. New York: Brazillier.

Minuchin, S. (1974) *Families and Family Therapy*. London: Tavistock Publications.

Ornstein, R.E. (1975) *The Psychology of Consciousness*. San Francisco: W.H. Freeman.

Pentony, P. (1981) *Models of Influence in Psychotherapy*. New York: Free Press.

Rieff, P. (1968) *The Triumph of the Therapeutic*. New York: Harper Torchbooks.

Rogers, C. (1975) *Client-Centred Therapy*. London: Constable.

Rogers, C.R. (1980) *A Way of Being*. Boston: Houghton Mifflin.

Rose, S. (1993) 'Child sacrifice: projective Christianity.' *Anima: The Journal of Human Experience 20*, 1, 12.

Smith, J., Osman, C. and Goding, M. (1990) 'Reclaiming the emotional aspects of the therapist-family system.' *Australian and New Zealand Journal of Family Therapy 11*, 3, 140–6.

Stagoll, B. (1991) 'Adelaide conversations: echoes that resound.' *Australian and New Zealand Journal of Family Therapy 12*, 2, 85–9.

Stewart, W. (1992) *An A–Z of Counselling Theory and Practice*. London: Chapman and Hall.

Strachey, J. (1965) *New Introductory Lectures to Psychoanalysis*. New York: Norton.

Tart, C. (ed) (1976) *Transpersonal Psychologies*. New York: Harper and Rowe.

Waldegrave, C.T. (1990) 'Just counselling.' *Dulwich Centre Newsletter: Social Justice and Family Therapy 1*.

Walters, M., Carter, B., Papp, P. and Silverstein, O. (1988) *The Invisible Web*. New York: Guilford.

Watts, A. (1975) *The Way of Zen*. New York: Vintage.

Watzlawick, P., Weakland, J.H. and Fisch, R. (1974) *Change: Principles of Problem Formation and Problem Resolution*. New York: Norton.

Whitaker, C. and Napier, A. (1978) *The Family Crucible*. New York: Harper and Row.

Wilhelm, R. (1967) *The I Ching or Book of Changes*. Princeton, New Jersey: Princeton University Press.

Williams, H. (1979) *The Joy of God*. New York: Penguin.

Wood, R.E. (1969) *Martin Buber's Ontology: An Analysis of I and Thou*. Evanston, IL: Northwestern University Press.

Winnicott, D.W. (1965) *The Maturational Processes and the Facilitating Environment*. London: Hogarth Press.

Index